The
One
Minute
H*(or so)*ealer

Also by Dana Ullman, M.P.H.

Books

Essential Homeopathy (New World Library, 2002)

The Steps to Healing: Wisdom from the Sages, the Rosemarys, and the Times (Hay House, 1999)

Homeopathy A–Z (Hay House, 1999)

Everybody's Guide to Homeopathic Medicine (with Stephen Cummings, M.D.) (Jeremy Tarcher/Putnam, 1997)

The Consumer's Guide to Homeopathy (Jeremy Tarcher/Putnam, 1996)

Homeopathic Medicines for Children and Infants (Jeremy Tarcher/Putnam, 1992)

Discovering Homeopathy (North Atlantic Books, 1991)

Homeopathic Family Medicine (an ebook published by www.homeopathic.com <http://www.homeopathic.com/>, updated bi-monthly)

Audiocassette

Homeopathic Healing (Sounds True, 1995)

The
One
Minute
(or so)
Healer

500 Simple Ways to Heal Yourself Naturally

Dana Ullman, M.P.H.

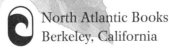

North Atlantic Books
Berkeley, California

Published by   and
North Atlantic Books   Homeopathic Educational Services
P.O. Box 12327   2124 Kittredge Street
Berkeley, California 94712   Berkeley, California 94704

Cover Design: Suzanne Albertson. *Illustrations:* John Holmquist. Acupressure graphics: Michael Reed Gach, Ph.D., Acupressure Institute, Berkeley, CA.

Printed in Canada.

The One-Minute (or so) Healer: 500 Simple Ways To Heal Yourself Naturally is sponsored by the Society for the Study of Native Arts and Sciences, a nonprofit educational corporation whose goals are to develop an educational and crosscultural perspective linking various scientific, social, and artistic fields; to nurture a holistic view of arts, sciences, humanities, and healing; and to publish and distribute literature on the relationship of mind, body, and nature.

The author of this book does not dispense medical advice or prescribe the use of any technique as a form of treatment for physical or medical problems without the advice of a physician, either directly or indirectly. The intent of the author is only to offer information of a general nature to help you in your quest for emotional and spiritual well-being. In the event you use any of the information in this book for yourself, which is your constitutional right, the author and the publisher assume no responsibility for your actions.

First published by Hay House in 2000. Portions of this work were originally published as part of the book *The One Minute or so Healer* by Dana Ullman, published by G.P. Putnam's Sons, New York, New York, © 1991.

Library of Congress Cataloging-in-Publication Data
Ullman, Dana.
    The one-minute (or so) healer : 500 simple ways to heal yourself naturally / by Dana Ullman.
        p. cm.
    ISBN 1-55643-494-4 (paperback)
    1. Alternative medicine. 2. Naturopathy. 3. Self-care, Health. I.
Title: One-minute or so healer. II. Title.
    R733 .U455 2004
    615.5'35–dc22
                                        200302508

1 2 3 4 5 6 7 8 9 TRANS 09 08 07 06 05 04

contents

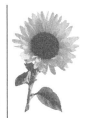

Acknowledgments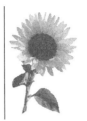

I can acknowledge people who have contributed to this book in a minute, but simply listing their names hardly seems adequate. I can and will acknowledge them throughout my lifetime. These people have not simply contributed to this book; they have contributed to me and my life . . . and now to you, the reader.

There are innumerable people who have planted in me seeds of knowledge, experience, insight, and wonder. I cannot name them all in a minute. Instead, I wish to acknowledge my various friends and colleagues who have given me specific feedback on different stages of this manuscript. These people are: Lynn Fraley, R.N., Dr.P.H.; James Gordon, M.D.; Ben Hole, M.D.; Sandra McLanahan, M.D.; Carolyn Reuben, C.A.; Michael Schmidt, D.C.; Jim Spira, Ph.D.; Richard Solomon, M.D.; Janet Zand Marcus, L.Ac., O.M.D.; Metece Riccio-Politi; Mary Marlowe; Alain Jean-Mairet; Mandy Lonsdale; Lani Hnatiuk; and Nancy Siciliana.

My editor for the first edition of this book, Donna Zerner, deserves a special thank you for her editing skills, her ideas, and her consistent and persistent vision of what this book could and should be. At times, I had disturbing side effects from her surgical editing, but my words and I have survived to tell the story.

John Holmquist, this book's illustrator, put my cartoon concepts into visual form. He didn't simply use my ideas, but infused many of his own in an artistic and humorous fashion.

I also want to thank my friend and colleague Michael Reed Gach, Ph.D., for letting me use the acupressure graphics used in select chapters of this book.

A special thanks to Richard Grossinger and Lindy Hough of North Atlantic Books for keeping this book alive and kicking.

Heartfelt thanks must also be given to my wife, Clare Ullman. Her ability to withstand my sense of humor at all hours of the day and night is truly Herculean. Always giving feedback on my bedside personality, she has helped me refine my healing and loving abilities. My son, Jacob, is my best audience. I thank him for his primordial laughter and for encouraging me to get in touch with my inner child and my inner adult.

introduction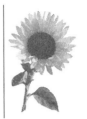

Becoming a healer in one minute is really no big deal. You've actually been working at healing longer than you think. Thousands of years of survival training have been built into your genes. From the moment of conception up to this very instant, every cell of your body has actively and continually defended itself against microbes, environmental assaults, and all types of stress. Perhaps most wonderful of all, your body has defended itself against you and the ravages you have inflicted on it.

Occasionally, of course, you need some help in healing. At times, you learn a technique or two to heal yourself; and at other times, you may go to a health expert.

This book will help you with the first choice. It will increase your knowledge of what you can do to help the expert healer inside you do its work. The premise of this book is: *If you take your disease lying down, you are apt to stay that way.*

Before Using One-Minute Strategies, Consider This

Many of you may have rushed to the chapters dealing with

specific one-minute strategies before reading this introduction. What's the hurry? As comedian Lily Tomlin once said, "For fast relief, slow down." Although it's natural to want to make it stop hurting as quickly as you can, it is important, sometimes even necessary, to *understand* healing in order to make it happen most effectively. This is not meant to make you feel guilty if you jumped to chapters that describe the one-minute strategies; it is simply to say that it is sometimes useful to read a book's introduction in order to get some insights on how to use the work most effectively.

Franz Kafka once wrote, "To write prescriptions is easy, but to come to an understanding with people is hard." Likewise, to take a vitamin, herb, or homeopathic medicine is simple, but to come to a real understanding of what is wrong with you and what you can do on a deeper level to make it right is more difficult. Before rushing off to do one or more of the one-minute strategies, I want to encourage you to read *The Steps to Healing,* a companion book to this one. This isn't meant to be a crass promotion for one of my other books; it is my encouragement to you to consider learning about the healing process and how to best augment it.

The book you have in your hands right now is full of specific techniques for initiating healing, while *The Steps to Healing* will describe the various steps and ground rules that allow healing to occur.

Now that I've said that, let's talk about this book.

Between 10 and 30 different strategies are offered for each condition. You are not expected or even encouraged to use all of them to heal your ailment (see Step #20 in *The Steps to Healing:* "Obsession with Health Can Be Sickening"). Try using a few of them one day, and a few more the next day until you feel better.

The one-minute strategies come from both Eastern and Western cultures and from ancient and modern traditions. Some strategies are part of folk medicine, some are a part of the cutting edge of contemporary medicine, and some will become an integral part of 21st-century healing.

Using "Unconventional" Methods

Some of the strategies recommended in this book are presently considered by the medical establishment to be "unconventional" or "unproven." Yet, many of them have been used for a considerably longer time than modern medical treatments; indeed, some have been used for thousands of years. The term *unconventional* is also dependent on where you are in the world. In many places, the use of herbs has always been considered completely conventional. In the Far East, acupuncture and acupressure are totally accepted, while our conventional medicine—encompassing the use of Cesarean-section births and artificial hearts—is not.

What is considered unconventional therapy today may

be mainstream tomorrow, and what is considered conventional medicine today may be tomorrow's quackery. This isn't a prediction; this is the evolution of medicine and science. Ultimately, the words *medicine* and *science* should be thought of as verbs, not nouns, for they are always changing, growing, and transforming.

Physicians too often overestimate the risks and underestimate the value of using unconventional therapies. At the same time, they tend to overestimate the value and underestimate the risks of conventional therapies. A healthy scientific attitude toward these presently unaccepted treatments is to maintain an open mind ... but not such an open mind that one's brain falls out.

On the other hand, it is important to seek conventional medical care when appropriate. If you have a potentially serious problem or recurring symptoms that are not remedied by the strategies recommended in this book, you should definitely get professional help immediately.

Ultimately, a collaborative approach that integrates natural and conventional treatment for healing is the best way to make it happen.

Using This Book

The One-Minute (or so) Healer provides specific strategies to help you heal yourself. Just as doctors "practice" medicine, you have to "practice" healing yourself. It is often necessary to experiment with one healing strategy or another, or a group of strategies. Such is the adventure of practicing healing and practicing life.

Although some people who have never tried or have rarely used natural therapies may feel uncomfortable with them, it is reassuring to know that natural healing strategies are generally safer and have been used for a considerably longer period of time than conventional medical treatments.

Have fun with these various healing strategies. Learning to utilize herbs with all their unusual textures and pungent fragrances is an enjoyable and empowering experience; pretend that you're a primitive medicine man or woman using herbal wisdom that has been passed on for generations in your tribe, or a shaman learning the secret language of body and soul. Discovering the safety and often rapid effectiveness of homeopathic medicines is very exciting, as is the detective work sometimes necessary to figure out the exact remedy to take for a particular set of symptoms. All of the strategies, from food choices to breathing exercises, will give you a sense of healthy control and connection to your body that is simply impossible to get from popping a laboratory-created pill.

This book is not intended to provide detailed information about every type of natural therapy. The books listed in the Recommended Resources section at the end of this book will help you learn more about the healing strategies that appeal to you.

Most of the suggested remedies are available at health food stores and select pharmacies. To help you find local sources of these products, you may want to contact health practitioners in your area who specialize in natural healing.

You are now ready to embark on the adventure of using these one-minute (or so) strategies for health and healing. Enjoy the process, and by the way, if you find that some of the strategies are taking longer than 60 seconds (it just might happen!), just put your stopwatch away, relax, and realize that your inner doctor has more patience than you know.

1 Acne

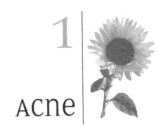

> *"Minds, like bodies, will often fall into a pimpled, ill-conditioned state from mere excess of comfort."*
> —CHARLES DICKENS

Carol Burnett once said, "Adolescence is just one big walking pimple." Although acne is an all-too-common problem for teenagers, adults experience it as well. Acne is one of those conditions that isn't physically painful or even physically discomforting; however, it certainly is a blow to the ego. Acne can turn a pretty face into a battlefield, where it looks like bombs have exploded, soldiers are bleeding, and no side is winning. It's easy to feel that acne is nature's revenge against the beauty of adolescence.

The good news is that you'll grow out of acne . . . usually.

For those adults who have acne, it can be even more embarrassing than for adolescents. The silver lining here is that people may think that you're a teenager!

On a more serious side, it's important to realize that skin symptoms do not necessarily indicate a skin disease. Skin symptoms are most likely internal problems that are manifesting on the skin. The skin is considered the third kidney—it is another organ of elimination that the body deploys to externalize oils and other matter not excreted from the body in the urine or stool. Because acne is more of an internal problem, it manifests through external symptoms, so it is not enough to simply wash your face regularly. Treating skin problems is an inside job.

Furthermore, you should be careful applying the various conventional external acne medications, for they can irritate the skin and suppress the external symptoms and create more serious internal ones.

It is also important to remember that having acne isn't all bad. Texture may be "in" this year or next. If, however, you do not want this to be your fashion statement, try these strategies.

Clean up your act. Hygiene is important, and you can benefit from washing your face two or three times a day. However, more frequent scrubbing can wash away important oils from the skin that help to lubricate it. If you use makeup, make certain to wash it off every night.

Too clean is too much. Avoid using soaps that dry out the skin or that cause any redness. Do not use alcohol as an astringent because it tends to dry out your skin too much. Witch hazel solutions are more effective astringents.

An herbal wash. Take the tincture of myrrh, dilute it in a small bowl of water, and use a swab of cotton to wipe your face. Myrrh's antiseptic and astringent properties can both treat and prevent acne.

Naturally antiseptic and drying. Tea tree oil is a powerful natural antiseptic and drying agent. Apply it directly to the skin wherever it is oily or where there are pimples. However, some people can develop an allergic reaction to this herbal remedy, so you may want to do a small patch test first. It is recommended to use products with 15 percent tea tree oil.

Steam those pimples out. Give yourself a facial steam bath. Place chamomile flowers or sage leaves in a bowl of water that has just finished boiling, and place a towel around your head. Create a mini-steambath for your face. For people who want a stronger herbal steambath, use tea tree oil, but be careful about using too much of this powerful, natural antiseptic (an alternative to using this herb in a steambath is to apply tea tree oil directly to the acne).

Oil's well does not always end well. Avoid oil-based cosmetics because they tend to clog skin pores. Cosmetic-induced acne is a common problem for many women. Look for cosmetics labeled "noncomodegenic."

Your hair is contagious. Keep hair off your face with a comb or brush. Wash your hair at least every second or third day.

To squeeze or not to squeeze. Most pimples should not be squeezed because a pimple is an inflammation, and you can cause infection by breaking it open. Worse still, squeezing them can sometimes scar you. However, if you are desperate and want at least some temporary improvement in your facial skin, use a hot, clean cloth or tissue to soften the pimple. This will allow you to break the pimple open with gentle pressure (the more pressure you have to use, the more likely you are to damage facial skin).

Supplement yourself. Vitamin A (25,000 IU daily), vitamin B complex (100 mg, 3 times/day), vitamin E (200–400 IU daily), and zinc (30–60 mg daily) are worthwhile supplements. Vitamin A can be used in an ointment, cream, or pill.

Good fats. Essential fatty acids (flaxseed oil, evening primrose oil, or borage oil are excellent sources) help keep skin soft and smooth and can dissolve fatty deposits that block skin pores. Take essential fatty acids daily.

Avoid drug abuse. Several prescription drugs, including many types of contraceptive pills and corticosteroids, can cause or aggravate acne.

Garbage inside, garbage outside. Acne can be affected by the food you eat. Although no foods have been proven to cause acne in all sufferers, some people observe reactions to milk products, nuts, fats, fried and oily foods, and chocolate.

Emotional garbage inside, emotional garbage outside. Emotions may be eating at you, literally. Emotional turmoil can disturb digestive and endocrine functions, leading to inefficient digestion of oils and to a potential increase in skin oils. The first step to deal with any emotional problem is to acknowledge it. Don't deny these emotions, but don't let them get the best of you either. Next, express what you are feeling; don't suppress it.

Face relaxation. Research has shown that people with acne have higher levels of anxiety and anger than other people do. However, this research didn't discern if the anxiety and anger led to the acne, or if the acne led to anxiety and anger. In any case, it is worthwhile to do something so that these emotions don't take a more serious toll on your health or on your face. Relaxation exercises may help you take greater control of your anxiety and irritability, rather than vice versa. Consider meditation, progressive relaxation, breathing exercises, or yoga. But don't try to do all these at the same time, since such efforts will lead to even more anxiety!

There is a real difference between cosmic beauty and cosmetic beauty. Everyone has his or her own inner beauty. Once you truly recognize this, you'll project it and appear to be even more beautiful.

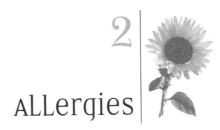

ALLergies

"The heart that is soonest awake to the flowers is always the first to be touched by the thorns."
—THOMAS MOORE

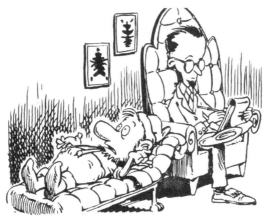

Sneezy has had a serious identity crisis ever since his allergies were cured.

[These strategies will primarily focus on the treatment of allergies with respiratory symptoms. If you have other symptoms of allergy, such as Asthma, Constipation, Diarrhea, Ear Infections, Fatigue, Headache, Indigestion, or Nausea, see the appropriate chapter.]

Freedom from allergies is literally nothing to sneeze at. This freedom, however, is a distant dream for many allergy sufferers.

Allergies can be imprisoning. They can make it difficult for some people to go outside, and they can even make it impossible to go for a simple walk in the country. Some allergy sufferers can't visit their friends who have pets, and many others can't eat their favorite foods.

Even the pleasures and benefits of exercise prove to be difficult, because some allergy sufferers' noses run more than they do. A runny or stuffy nose leads to mouth breathing, then a dry mouth, then less efficient breathing, and then less efficient overall functioning. A domino effect is set up, and the allergy sufferer is knocked down.

Conventional medical treatment for allergies usually consists of antihistamines, steroids, and desensitization shots. In stubborn cases, laser surgery may be utilized to vaporize mucus-forming nasal tissue. Be very careful of these treatments, however, since they all have side effects. Worst of all, these treatments may be the prelude to the most serious of all allergy treatments: cutting off the nose (not really, but these other treatments are almost as harmful to your sensitive nose).

Perhaps the greatest misunderstanding about allergies is the assumption that the allergen (the cat dander, the pollen, the house dust mite, or whatever) is the problem. Actually, the allergen is simply the trigger, while the allergic person's body is the loaded gun. Rather than just treating symptoms or avoiding the allergen, it is wise to take action to strengthen the body's own immune and defense system. Natural therapies that provide this more beneficial action help empty the loaded gun, or simply make it shoot blanks.

Unless you own shares of stock in Kleenex and don't mind purchasing it in bulk quantities, consider the following strategies. Some of these will strengthen your body and potentially reduce your allergies, while others will primarily reduce your exposure to the allergen.

Be breast-fed. Okay, this isn't really a one-minute strategy for you, but it is an effective strategy for your infant. Breast-feeding reduces the risk of getting allergies later in life.

Take a shower and wash your clothes more often. If you are carrying on your body and your clothes the pollen, cat dander, or other substances to which you are allergic, you may be continually reinfecting yourself.

Wash your pillow. One of the most common sources of allergies is dust mites that can inhabit the insides and outsides of a pillow. Although they will make their home in synthetic substances as easily as they will in down or foam, synthetic pillows have the advantage of being washable.

It is also a good idea to vacuum your bed (as strange as that may sound!) in order to get rid of this great breeding ground for dust mites, which are a very common source of allergies.

Dust be gone! Those dust mites and molds can hide any-where—in carpeting, drapes, and even teddy bears. Vacuum frequently, don't neglect washing the drapes, and avoid stuffed animals unless they have been recently washed.

Dry out. Use dehumidifiers and air conditioners to dry out humid rooms. Molds and dust mites tend to grow there.

Ventilate your car's air conditioner. If you plan to use the air conditioner, run it with the windows open for five minutes before getting into the car. Also, there are some products that decontaminate your air conditioner, so try to do this once a year. You should also consider deconta-minating your humidifier with one-half cup of liquid bleach to a gallon of water—as much as once a week if used fre-quently.

Get a pet alligator. Although many people are allergic to various kinds of animals, it is rare to be allergic to rep-tiles or fish. Consider getting a pet lizard, frog, fish, or alligator (just kidding on the latter). Such an acquisition won't necessarily cure your allergy, but it will give you a friend to love and cherish, which may be at least somewhat therapeutic.

Don't drink and sneeze. Alcohol can aggravate an allergy because it causes swelling of the mucous membranes. Don't drink and sneeze, since you may blow yourself away.

Don't mix antihistamines and grapefruit juice. Grapefruit juice actually has the capacity to inhibit the breakdown of antihistamines in your blood, thereby making this drug too powerful and sometimes too toxic. Choose one or the other.

Put the pressure on. Acupressure points at the base of the nostrils and in the indentations of the eye sockets, on either side of where the bridge of the nose meets the ridge of the eyebrows, help open the sinuses to clear your nose.

Use your thumbs to apply pressure for three to five seconds, let up, and then reapply the pressure.

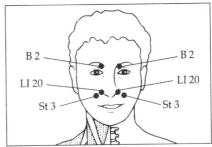

Eat your honey. To be more precise, eat your *local* honey. There are very small doses of pollen in honey that sometimes can help "immunize" the allergy sufferer to the pollen. There are also various pollen products on the market, although the best results will come from pollen grown as close to your home as possible. Local honey has homeopathic doses of various pollen in it which then helps prevent and heal some people who have respiratory allergies.

Vitamins to blow your allergies away. Take 500–1,000 mg of vitamin C three times a day, and 400 IUs of vitamin E twice a day. Also, take 400 mg of quercetin (a natural flavonoid and antioxidant) twice a day between meals, and 50 mg of bromelain (they usually come together in the same pill).

Sting those allergies. Research has found that the freeze-dried herb stinging nettle *(Urtica dioica)* has significant effects on upper respiratory allergy symptoms. Freeze-dried preparations of stinging nettle are available in capsule form in quality health food and herb stores. Take one or two capsules every two to four hours. It is not recommended to apply the fresh stinging nettle directly to the nose (it even hurts to think about this!).

Skunk cabbage is a great remedy for hay fever. Make an herbal tea of it, and drink a cup at least twice a day.

Miso your allergies. Miso soup, which is made from fermented, aged soybean puree, contains enzymes that aid digestion and can relieve symptoms of allergy.

Milk is* not *for every body, despite what the ads say. More people are allergic to milk and milk products than to any other food. Nature made cows' milk for calves, not humans. Avoid it as much as humanly possible.

Pollinate yourself homeopathically. If you have hay fever, you can temporarily alleviate your symptoms with a combination of homeopathic medicines made from flowers that create commonly irritating pollens. Research published in the British medical journal *The Lancet* showed this to be a very effective treatment. Various homeopathic companies have allergy and hay fever products that contain common pollens. Take this medicine every four hours while you have symptoms, and stop once the symptoms have dissipated. If you don't notice results within 48 hours, seek a more individualized homeopathic medicine after looking in a homeopathic guidebook, or try another strategy.

Take "a hair of the dog that bit you." If you are allergic to house dust mites (a very common allergy!), take a homeopathic dose of it *(House dust mite 30)* four times a day when you have allergy symptoms.

Make scents. Aromatherapy recommends placing one drop of the essential oil of lavender on your cheekbones at least twice a day.

Visualize being close to or even touching that substance to which you are allergic. Picture yourself responding to it without any allergy symptoms. Think or say aloud, "Every day and in every way I am able to touch _____ in a normal and healthy way." Although this exercise can initially cause allergic symptoms, it can ultimately help reduce them.

Make peace with whatever you are allergic to. Just because you are allergic to cats doesn't mean that you have to hate them. You can still appreciate these wonderful feline creatures . . . at a distance. This may not rid you of your allergy or other symptoms, but it certainly works better than cursing the cat, the pollen, or the mold.

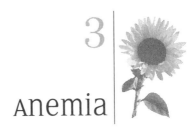

3

anemia

*"An ounce of blood is worth more than
a pound of friendship."*
—SPANISH PROVERB

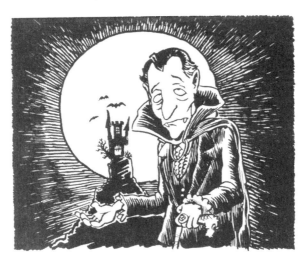

Anemic people create lethargic vampires.

People with anemia may have the "blahs," or in the language of 1950s television, they have "iron-poor blood." Besides being easily fatigued, anemic individuals have pale complexions, dizziness, headaches, brittle nails, and even depression. Anemia can also lead to mental exhaustion and dullness, making reading a tad more difficult (good thing this book is useful for people with short attention spans!).

Anemia is the reduction in the oxygen-carrying capacity of the blood. It is a type of suffocation that the blood experiences as the result of inadequate nutrition, a loss of blood due to injury or disease, or the result of certain diseases such as sickle cell anemia, in which the body's red blood cells are being destroyed.

People who are more likely to have anemia are those who may have iron deficiencies, including:

- women, because they menstruate;
- pregnant and lactating women, because of their increased nutritional requirements;
- people with gastrointestinal disorders, because internal bleeding leads to blood loss;
- strict vegetarians who do not eat any meat or dairy products and who do not know vegetarian sources of iron;
- aspirin takers, because this drug can cause internal bleeding;

- children who are in a growth phase; and
- the elderly, due to poor iron absorption.

Just because you fit in any of the above categories does not mean that you should take iron supplements, because these supplements can lead to an overdose of iron. This can particularly be a problem for pregnant women.

Remember, anemia isn't a disease; it's a *symptom* of disease. It is a sign and signal that the body isn't able to oxygenate its blood adequately. In the meantime, or after seeing your doctor, the following strategies are relatively easy and can be performed quite bloodlessly. However, if your condition does not resolve within a couple of weeks, consider medical care to identify the underlying cause of this condition. In any case, avoid vampires. Additional loss of blood may aggravate your condition.

Pass on the coffee, tea, and soda. Avoid coffee and black tea, especially one hour before or after a meal, since they can interfere with iron absorption from 40 to 95 percent! Coffee and tea ultimately drain you because they provide short-term energy but create longer-term fatigue. Also, avoid sodas, since they contain excessive amounts of phosphates that can interfere with iron absorption. Other phosphate-laden products include beer, ice cream, cheese, candy bars, baked goods, and EDTA (a common preservative).

Avoid the iron scuds. Chocolate, blueberries, and summer squash all contain chemicals called oxalates, which interfere with iron absorption. Avoid these foods that shoot iron down.

Eat "red" things, which can nourish your red blood. Eat liver (if organic), cherries and cherry juice, eggplant, raisins, prunes, and the seaweed dulse. Raw liver extracts are available in pill form and are particularly useful because they contain healthy amounts of iron, folic acid, and vitamin B_{12}.

Pump iron. Other foods that have a lot of iron in them are sea vegetables (dulse, nori, and kelp); white meat chicken; dark meat turkey; blackstrap molasses; pumpkin seeds; sunflowers; oysters; eggs; garbanzo beans; brewers yeast; and green leafy vegetables (especially kale, beet greens, and chard). Eat nails if you're an anemic robot; eat foods with iron in them if you're an anemic human.

Cook in iron. Cook your food in cast iron, and you will receive trace amounts in your food. How simple!

Take iron supplements ... carefully. Because iron supplements can interfere with zinc and magnesium absorption and destroy vitamin E stores in the body, this vitamin should be taken with care. You should not take an iron supplement in larger dose than the recommended daily allowance (between 10 and 30 mg) unless you're under medical supervision.

Vitamins C and E promote iron absorption. Take 500 mg of vitamin C twice a day, and 200 IU of vitamin E.

Beauty and the Bs. Proper amounts of folic acid and B_{12} are also important for absorption of iron. It is recommended to take .5–1 mg of folic acid and 1,000–2,000 mcg of B_{12} daily.

There's iron in them-there herbs. Several herbs are rich in iron, and when made into a tea, they provide a healthy amount of iron. A combination of the following herbs is recommended: nettles, dandelion leaves, and yellowdock root. Nettle (also commonly called "stinging nettle") is particularly iron-rich. The dried (nonstinging) herb is readily available in health food and herb stores. The fresh nettles can be steamed and taste like spinach, but they're tastier. Just be very careful in handling them in this fresh state, since their spines can cause a sharp and burning irritation. When making a tea, you can choose to use just one or all three herbs. It is rarely necessary to drink more than two cups a day, and don't do so for more than two weeks at a time.

Eat foods with copper in them. Copper helps the body assimilate the iron in foods. Foods that have copper in them are organ meats, seafood, nuts, legumes, and molasses.

Expect to sink if you over-zinc. Overconsumption of zinc supplements can lead to copper deficiency, which can then cause anemia.

Don't overdo fiber or calcium. Fiber acts as a laxative, and too much of it can help wash iron out of your body before it gets absorbed. Also, some grains have in their bran a type of acid called phytic acid, which interferes with iron absorption. High calcium intake inhibits iron absorption, too.

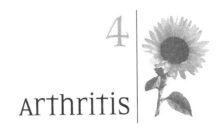

Arthritis

*"I don't deserve this award, but I have arthritis,
and I don't deserve that either."*
—Jack Benny

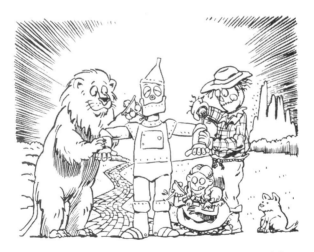

How arthritic stiffness is treated in the Land of Oz.

Sir William Osler, considered to be the "Father of Modern Medicine," once said, "When an arthritis patient walks in the front door, I feel like leaving by the back door." And it is no wonder that it pained Dr. Osler to try to treat arthritic patients—there is little that conventional medicine offers these individuals. The lucky ones get temporary relief along with drug side effects; the unlucky ones only get the side effects.

Some arthritic patients experience such constant pain that they'd like to follow Dr. Osler out the back door or simply have an out-of-body experience, leaving their pain behind.

The word *arthritis* means "inflammation of a joint," and there are various ways in which people experience this. There are dozens of kinds of arthritis: osteoarthritis, rheumatoid arthritis, gout, systemic lupus, and bursitis, to name just a few. The good news is that arthritis will rarely kill you. The bad news is that the stiffness that sufferers experience can make them feel as though rigor mortis has set in early.

Osteoarthritis is the most common type of arthritis. Sometimes called the "wear and tear" variety of arthritis, osteoarthritis is thought to be a natural result of aging. This is just a theory; however, as evidenced by the 93-year-old man from Chicago who developed osteoarthritis in his left knee. When his doctor told him that it was a result of aging, the wise man remarked, "My other knee is 93 years old, too, and it don't hurt a bit."

There are other factors besides aging that precipitate osteoarthritis. Likewise, each type of arthritis has numerous influences that increase or decrease the chances of getting it. It is known, for instance, that women experience most types of arthritis two to eight times as often as men (gout and ankylosing spondylitis are the exceptions). Sorry, ladies, but sex-change operations are not therapeutically effective.

Here, however, are some strategies that may help you.

Use it, or you lose it. Range-of-motion exercises are very important in increasing circulation and reducing stiffness. Although one should avoid exercising a joint that is currently inflamed or "hot," these joints can be gently moved along their range of motion. Swimming is a particularly good exercise for people with arthritis. Although jogging is not associated with degenerative joint disease, you might consider walking as an alternative form of exercise if you experience any joint pain during or after jogging. Don't overdo any exercise, but don't underdo it either. Try to exercise 15 to 20 minutes a day, five days a week.

Avoid arthritis "cooperators." Some evidence suggests that certain foods can aggravate an arthritic condition. Although such foods are not thought to "cause" arthritis, they may "cooperate" with it and make it worse. Experiment by avoiding foods from the nightshade family, including tomatoes, eggplant, peppers (except black pepper), and potatoes (except for potato juice—explained further on). Tobacco is also a member of the nightshade family that can aggravate arthritis. Milk, fats, and citrus fruits are other possible cooperators. As an experiment, avoid, or at least significantly reduce, ingesting them.

The danger of conventional drugs. The most common conventional drugs used in arthritis treatment are non-steroidal anti-inflammatory drugs (NSAIDs), including aspirin and ibuprofen. While these drugs may provide temporary relief of pain, they may aggravate the person's arthritis by inhibiting cartilage formation and accelerating cartilage destruction. Their frequent and long-term use can also cause various other serious side effects. People with rheumatoid arthritis or those who take aspirin frequently may benefit from taking 500 mg of vitamin C per day because they tend to be deficient in it.

Cut yourself down to size. Avoid wearing high heels, which tend to place excessive pressure on certain joints and aggravate your condition. They can also hurt your posture.

Something to straighten you out and loosen you. Researchers don't fully understand why, but sex—with or without a partner—has been found to relieve arthritic pain. This does not have to be a one-minute strategy.

Apply some herbal heat. Cayenne pepper is known to contain a painkilling chemical called capsaicin. There are now some over-the-counter drugs as well as some herbal products that are primarily composed of capsaicin. Apply it externally directly to and around the source of pain. Ideally, use a standardized cream with 0.025%–0.075% capsaicin. Expect your initial applications to produce a burning sensation.

Let herbs help you bend in the wind. Make an herbal tea with equal parts of alfalfa, chickweed, and yucca.

Claw away at it. Cat's claw contains powerful antioxidants that fight free radicals and help relieve joint pain and inflammation. Pregnant women should avoid taking this herbal remedy.

Glucosamine what? Glucosamine is a natural substance found in high concentration in the body's cartilage and joints. Although it doesn't exhibit significant anti-inflammatory or analgesic properties, it provides structural support to the joints and helps relieve the pain and discomfort in many people suffering from arthritis. Consider taking 500 mg three times a day, preferably on an empty stomach, but if irritation occurs, take it with food. By the way, most of the best research on people with arthritis has been with glucosamine sulfate; consider using this type of glucosamine first. By the way, some sources suggest that people with a heart condition should avoid taking this supplement.

Spice up your life. The popular herb/spice turmeric contains a yellow pigment called curcumin, which has very potent anti-inflammatory activity. It has been found to be useful for people suffering from rheumatoid arthritis. Take 400 mg three times a day. Typically, it is sold with bromelain, which is a mixture of enzymes that help the body absorb curcumin.

All's well that ends boswellia. Boswellia is an herb that is extremely well known in Ayurvedic medicine. Laboratory research has shown that it can help block certain hormonelike chemicals and immune cells involved in the inflammation of arthritis. It is generally recommended to take one pill three times a day (each pill should be standardized to contain 150 mg of boswellic acids).

MSM to the rescue. MSM (Methylsulfonylmethane) is a nutritional supplement containing sulphur that seems to have a powerful effect on inhibiting pain impulses along nerves, thereby acting as an anti-inflammatory and analgesic. It is thought to be particularly useful for people with osteoarthritis. Consider using 750 mg three times a day. In order to minimize digestive complaints, it is best to take it with food. If taking MSM in a combination with glucosamine, take one with 500 mg of each. If you are on anticoagulants, consult with your doctor before using MSM.

Not just the Sam-e old thing. Sam-e is not a misspelling; it stands for S-adenosylmethionine, which is a form of amino acid. It produces a similar anti-inflammatory effect as ibuprofen, but this more natural substance has been shown to rebuild cartilage. The problem is that it is more expensive than most supplements (but less than many drugs!). Take 400 mg twice a day for two weeks, and then 200 mg twice a day as a maintenance dose. If you have manic-depressive illness, it is best not to take it.

Water yourself. Stimulate circulation in the affected areas by taking a hot shower or bath, and then turn on the cold water. Repeat the hot cycle, and then return to the cold. If your hands, knees, or feet are the primary sources of pain, you can simply place them in a tub or sink of hot and then cold water. Another alternative is to place a hot pack on a specific area and alternate with a cold pack. Try this at least twice a day.

Become an "opiate-like" substance addict. Research has shown that the brain creates beta-endorphins, which are opiate-like substances that naturally reduce pain. Research has also discovered that there are lower amounts of beta-endorphins in the blood of some arthritic sufferers. Physical exercises and relaxation exercises both have been found to increase these natural painkillers.

A need for kneading. It doesn't take a rocket scientist to know that massage is good for people with arthritis. For best results, avoid massaging directly on top of an inflamed joint. Instead, massage just above and below the joint.

Press a point near a joint. Press a pressure point that is near, but not on top of, the primary source of pain. You can find a good pressure point by feeling a slight crease in the skin (it will probably be tender). Press this point for three to five seconds, let up for a bit, and press it a couple more times in a similar manner. Some other good pressure points may be around (not directly on) nearby joints. Try to press firmly but not too hard. Breathe into it, and you will find that the pain lessens.

Cast castor oil on the pain. Make a castor oil pack, and place it on a joint where there is pain, but not when there's acute inflammation. To make it, pour three or four tablespoons of castor oil in a pan, heat the oil until it simmers, then saturate a flannel cloth with the oil. After you place this cloth on the affected joint, cover it with a larger towel and place an electric heating pad over it. Keep it in place for 30 to 60 minutes. This castor oil pack can be saved for future use by simply rolling up the cloth and placing it in a Ziploc bag.

Become a juice potato. An old folk remedy for arthritis is to drink raw potato juice. To make it, wash a potato (don't peel it), cut it into thin slices, place it in a glass of cold water, and leave it out overnight. Drink this water in the morning on an empty stomach. The lowly potato is known to have antiviral inhibitors and is rich in chlorogenic acid, which helps prevent cell mutations that lead to cancer. Whatever it is in potatoes that helps arthritic sufferers is yet to be found, but personal experience suggests that it can be helpful.

Fish oil can lubricate you. Research has recently shown that fish oil supplements have anti-inflammatory effects that may be helpful to arthritis sufferers. One important study showed beneficial effects when people took 15 capsules a day, although most people will probably experience benefits by taking four to eight capsules daily. Recent research has also suggested that extracts from the New Zealand green- lipped mussel, now available in supplement form, are particularly good for people with osteoarthritis and rheumatoid arthritis. Although this supplement may sound strange, would you rather suffer, or try something that might make you feel better?

Life should be a bowl of cherries. Some people report relief from arthritis symptoms after eating lots of cherries, especially sour cherries. Sour cherries contain antioxidants that inhibit the Cox-2 enzyme, which exacerbates arthritic inflammation.

Bejewel yourself in copper. People suffering from arthritis have been known to experience relief when they wear a copper bracelet. Although skeptics point to this treatment as a classic example of quackery, or simply the placebo effect, it is known that some people with arthritis have difficulty assimilating copper from the food they eat. Perhaps wearing a copper bracelet provides them with a subtle but biologically active source of this mineral. Lending further support to the use of copper, homeopathic physicians commonly prescribe microdoses of copper *(Cuprum metalicum)* to those people with arthritis who experience cramping pains in the joints and jerking or twitching of muscles.

Bee stings for arthritis? It is a well-known bit of folklore that beekeepers have a low incidence of arthritis. It is also known that one folk remedy for treating arthritis is getting stung by a bee. An easier way to try this remedy is to get a homeopathic dose of bee venom in *Apis mellifica* 6 or 30. This medicine is primarily helpful if you have arthritic pain that is similar to the type of pain that bee venom causes: burning pain, aggravated by heat, alleviated by cold or cool applications.

Could poison ivy be helpful? Actually, yes, but only homeopathic doses of it. Poison ivy, known as *Rhus tox* in homeopathy, is a very effective medicine if you have the "rusty gate" type of arthritis—that is, pain that is worse upon initial motion and reduced as you continue to move. If you have this pattern of symptoms, *Rhus tox* 6 or 30 may be helpful to you. If, however, your pain is increasingly aggravated by any type of motion and is not alleviated by continued motion, take *Bryonia* 6 or 30.

Are you too resistant to change? Is the stiffness in your character creating stiffness in your body? There's the story of two caterpillars who look up and notice a butterfly. One caterpillar says to the other: "You'll never get me up in one of those." Are you resisting any inevitable changes in your life? Loosen up. Say to yourself: "I expect change, and I will bend with it."

Dear, Dear Diary. Keep a diary of your symptoms. Look for patterns of what might aggravate the pain that you experience. Finding a pattern might not "cure" you, but it may help you avoid those things that trigger your pain syndrome. Also, recent research has found that simply writing about your experiences with arthritis has a therapeutic benefit. Write on!

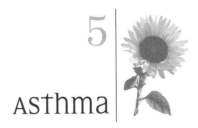

5

Asthma

*"I durst not laugh, for fear of opening
my lips and receiving the bad air."*
—from Shakespeare's *Julius Caesar*

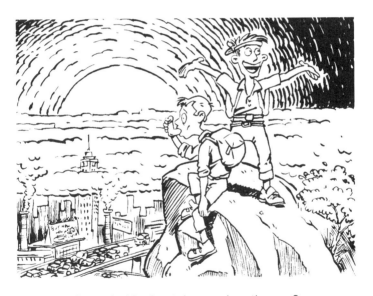

Doesn't this view take your breath away?

Some people say that the best treatment for people with asthma is "parent-ectomy." Although parents' smothering can certainly be an influence, there are other factors that predispose people to both breathlessness and asthma.

Asthma is primarily an allergic condition that can be triggered by various foods, preservatives, pollens, weeds, grasses, chemicals and fumes, the house dust mite, or tobacco. Emotional stress and vigorous exercise can also trigger an attack.

Just a couple of decades ago, few people died from asthma. However, deaths in children from asthma are growing at an alarming rate. One can't help but wonder if the powerful steroidal drugs that are used to control symptoms and that also suppress immune function play an important role in this death toll. Don't let this type of drug abuse hurt your family. Seek out alternatives. It *is* a matter of life and breath.

Having your breath taken away as the result of a romantic interlude is wonderful. However, if you're having your breath taken away at other times, too, consider these strategies.

Just don't sit there, relax! Feeling tense and anxious makes breathing more difficult. Being tense is like trying to untie a knot by pulling at both ends. Relax, and the knot almost unties itself. Progressive relaxation in which you first tense and then relax muscle groups is an effective way to achieve a heightened state of relaxation. Make sure to relax those shoulders; it's hard to breathe fully when your shoulders are up around your ears (it makes hearing more difficult, too).

Don't just sit there, move! Certain exercises that strengthen the lungs can be very helpful. Swimming is best, especially the breaststroke. Aerobic dancing has also been found to be helpful to asthmatics. Start all exercise programs slowly, take breaks when you feel a need for them, and don't overdo it. There were five gold medalists in the 1972 Olympics who suffered from asthma, so don't assume that asthma has to limit your ability to exercise.

Vacuum cleaning therapy. Perhaps the most common substance to trigger asthmatic breathing is the feces from the house dust mite. Vacuum as much as possible. Make certain to also vacuum the bed (and wash your pillows), since they can be prefect breeding grounds for dust mites. When you vacuum rigorously, it can become an aerobic exercise, which in itself is therapeutic. If, however, you are hypersensitive to dust, any type of vacuuming can trigger symptoms. For these people, it is recommended to have others do "vacuum therapy" while you sit back and practice relaxation therapy.

Give your skin the brush-off. Your skin is a third lung. It breathes and oxygenates you. Avoid covering your body with oil when you have respiratory problems, since you want to keep your third lung breathing freely. Take a loofah or any soft bristle brush and stimulate your skin.

Be cool. This one is easy ... turn the heat down. Many people with asthma have difficulty breathing in a heated room. Open a window, too, unless you're chilled by it; you'll want to avoid overly cold temperatures, because extremes of temperature can aggravate symptoms.

Humidify yourself. Humidifiers can help loosen the mucus that is blocking your breathing. You can potentiate the action of the humidifier by placing a teaspoon of eucalyptus, mullein, or thyme in a cold mist humidifier or vaporizer. Make sure to wash the humidifier after each use. If you don't have a humidifier, put the oil into a pot of steaming water, and place your face over the pot while you cover your head with a towel. Do this for as long as it feels good.

Preserve yourself by avoiding preservatives. Certain preservatives, particularly sulfites and MSG, can trigger an asthma attack. Sulfites are often put in wine, beer, dried fruit, and seafood. They are also put in salad bars to keep the vegetables looking fresh. MSG is a common ingredient in Chinese food. Ask to have your food prepared without it.

Breathergizing #1. Diaphragmatic breathing exercises your lungs and abdomen and helps give you a full breath. To make certain that you're doing it correctly, follow these instructions. Place your hands on your waist above the hips. Your fingers should slightly extend over the sides of your lower abdomen, and the thumb should slightly extend over the sides of your back. Focus your attention on how your hands move when you breathe. Proper diaphragmatic breathing is occurring when your hands are thrust out to each side, rather than primarily thrust forward.

Breathergizing #2. Practice expiratory breathing. This type of breathing is when you inspire normally, but exert slightly additional pressure during the exhalation. Don't push too hard. This breathing helps to dilate the bronchial passages. Do whatever visualization practices will augment this breathing exercise. For instance, imagine yourself pushing out the walls of a room. This may then give you more "room for breathing."

Breathergizing #3. Take a full breath through your nose. When you exhale, pronounce out loud the syllables "woo," "ee," and "ah" on separate exhalations. Pronounce each syllable for five or six seconds each. Gradually increase the length of your exhalations. After doing each syllable at least twice, observe your breath, and see if you are now taking deeper, fuller breaths.

Bolster your breathing. Lie on the floor and place a bolster or large pillow under your upper back, just below the shoulders. Your head should touch the floor. Slowly place your arms above your head; your chest will be lifted, and your back will be arched. Breathe fully into your chest and abdomen. Maintain this position for one to five minutes, but don't overstrain.

Do the cobra. The cobra is a yoga posture that aids asthma sufferers by opening their breathing passages. You begin by lying on your abdomen and placing your hands palms down under your shoulders. While inhaling, raise your head and then your chest, using your back muscles and your hands to support you. Try to raise yourself near the point at which your arms are not bent. Hold this position until you wish to exhale, and then slowly relax yourself back to the floor. Repeat this exercise at least five times.

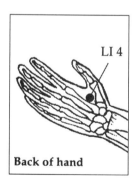

LI 4

Back of hand

Your lungs are in your hands. There is an acupressure point right in your hands that will provide healing energy to the lungs. It is in the web of your hands between the thumb and second finger. You may notice that this area is very sensitive to pressure; this a sign that it needs to be pressed. Do so for at least five seconds, and repeat it several times. Another good acupressure point to improve lung function is the web between your big toe and your second toe.

Supplement your breathing. Research has shown that 100–150 mg of vitamin B_6 is helpful to people with asthma. You might also want to supplement this supplement with 1,000 mg of vitamin C, 200–400 IU of vitamin E, and 1–4 mcg of B_{12} (the latter is especially good for sulfite-sensitive people).

Put spice in your life. Various pungent foods and spices have bronchodilating effects that can relieve symptoms of allergy. Of specific value are onions, garlic, chili peppers, horseradish, and mustard.

It's coffee time. Coffee also has bronchodilating effects. Research has shown that two cups of brewed coffee can relieve symptoms of asthma in one or two hours for up to six hours. Although the medicinal use of coffee may seem surprising to some people involved in natural medicine, we must remember that coffee, like every other herb, can be therapeutic in one dose and poisonous in another. Don't use this strategy if you are sensitive to coffee's other effects.

Is it a drug, or is it an herb? Ephedrine is a very popular drug that was once commonly given to people with asthma. Although this drug improves breathing, it also had various side effects, including nervousness, insomnia, increased heart rate, and dizziness. Because of this, it is not as popular as it previously was. However, there is an herb called Ephedra (also called Ma Huang and Mormon Tea) which contains ephedrine in smaller, safer doses. Making a tea of Ephedra with a half ounce of the branches in one pint of water and drinking one or two cups provides the benefits of ephedrine without the side effects. You can also consider taking this herb in pill form. It should, however, be taken on a short-term basis only; and should not be taken by people with high blood pressure, insomnia, anxiety and restlessness, or prostate cancer.

Use a hair of the mite that bit you. Asthma is commonly the result of exposure to the house dust mite, a microscopic organism that grows on house dust. This is actually one of the most common allergens in the world, and some excellent research has shown that homeopathic doses of it (the 30th potency) are very effective in providing relief. Consider using it every four hours for no more than a couple of days at a time. Consider seeking professional homeopathic care for a "constitutional remedy" to potentially cure the underlying allergic condition, of which the asthma is but one part.

No smothering allowed. We all sometimes feel crowded, either physically or psychologically. While this doesn't bother some people, it can truly suffocate others. As they say in California, "Encourage others to respect your space." In other words, kindly tell people to avoid crowding you, either physically or with their expectations. At the same time, you might explore those characteristics in yourself that seek approval from others, that desire attention, and that want to be smothered by others.

Write on! Recent research has found that keeping a journal and writing about your asthma symptoms provides a therapeutic benefit, as compared with people who simply write about the mundane activities that they plan to do during the day.

Emotions allowed. Many people with asthma notice that attacks may be triggered when they bottle up their emotions. Allow yourself to feel whatever emotions you feel. Accept them and express them. The more they are bottled up inside you, the more they explode internally. Suppression of emotions can be enough to take your breath away.

Avoid cockroaches and chocolate. People with asthma are often allergic to cockroaches. Keep your house as clean as possible to discourage cockroaches from hanging around. Also, did you know that the FDA allows manufacturers a certain percentage by weight of cockroach parts in chocolate? It is apparently very difficult to keep these insects out of the chocolate vats (can you blame them?), so the best way to avoid cockroaches is to avoid chocolate. Strange, but true!

6

Bladder Infections (Cystitis)

"The length of a film should be directly related to the endurance of the human bladder."

—ALFRED HITCHCOCK

B ladder infections cause frequent, urgent, and painful urination. Although not usually a dangerous medical problem, any condition that reduces the relief involved in going to the bathroom, and the pleasure related to making love—and which actually causes pain from doing so—should be considered somewhat serious, if not by the doctor, then at least by the patient. Approximately half of all women get a bladder infection at least once in their life, and one in four women experiences repeated bladder infections. It's enough to really—uh, tick, that's it—tick you off.

Bladder infections are much more common in women than in men. One reason is because the woman's urethra, the tube connecting the bladder to the outside of the body, is only a half inch long, and this opening is so close to the anus that infection from nearby bacteria is relatively easy to come by.

However, only about 50 percent of bladder infections are the result of bacterial infection. Other factors that trigger a bladder infection include a *Candida* (fungal) infection or an allergic response to certain foods or drinks. Vigorous sex and certain perfumed soaps can also irritate the urethra and the bladder. It's ironic that getting "down and dirty" or getting "squeaky-clean" can create problems. Vibrations, either from riding a motorcycle or using a vibrator, can also irritate the bladder (gee, I know you're going to miss that motorcycle).

Antibiotics will not be helpful treatments, except in the case of bacterial infections. Because antibiotics can disrupt the balance of helpful vaginal bacteria, the inappropriate use of these drugs can cause a *Candida* infection. Get a culture to see if you have a bacterial infection, and also consider these strategies.

Drink up! Drink lots of fluid, but avoid coffee, black tea, caffeinated sodas, and alcohol, which can all aggravate your bladder. These beverages may taste good going in, but they can hurt coming out. Ouch. Try to drink at least eight glasses of water a day.

Take acid. Drink two or three glasses of unsweetened cranberry juice a day. This juice acidifies your urine and burns those bacteria or fungi out of your body. There are now capsules available that primarily consist of unsweetened cranberry juice (it will probably be easier to find this than the juice). Taking 500 mg of vitamin C three times a day also acidifies your urine. Some women report irritation from citrus fruits and spicy foods, so you may want to avoid them.

Clean up your act. Sit in a tub or basin of warm or hot water for 20 minutes. Put a half cup of white or apple cider vinegar in the water. No soap should be used. Make certain to keep your legs spread in order to cleanse the genital area. Repeat this in 2 hours, and again, 12 hours later.

Empty yourself. Try to empty your bladder as often as possible, at least every three or four hours during the day. Also, try to urinate just before having sex and especially immediately after.

Get cultured. Eat unsweetened yogurt, or drink miso soup at least once a day. Yogurt and miso provide helpful bacterial cultures to your body, which is particularly important if you are taking antibiotics.

Not so sweet. Bacteria thrive on sweet blood. Avoid keeping your blood sugar high by not eating too many sweets.

Be careful of hot pants. Tight pants or underwear not made from natural fibers don't allow adequate breathing. Yes, you *do* breathe down there, too (in fact, you breathe through every pore in your skin). Synthetic fibers create an environment more conducive to bladder infections. Stick to 100 percent cotton or silk.

Feeling the pressure? An ill-fitting diaphragm can press against the urethra and ultimately irritate the bladder. Wide-lipped diaphragms put less pressure on the urethra. Speaking of sex, make certain to engage in foreplay before making love (this shouldn't be a one-minute strategy). The woman should be adequately lubricated before the man inserts his penis. Also, the man should avoid scented condoms, since they may irritate the woman.

Don't wipe yourself out. When women urinate, they should wipe from front to back. Wiping from back to front could spread anal bacteria to the urethra.

Herbal soothers. The following herbs should be mixed together and made into a tea: marshmallow (not marshmallows!), barberry (not blueberries), or uva ursi (not *e pluribus unum!*), sage (not just any wise herb!), corn silk (not silk pajamas!), and horsetail (not the type that take you for a ride!). Place approximately one tablespoon of a mixture of these herbs per cup in boiling water, and let simmer for five minutes. When cool, drink one to three cups per day. If you prefer taking a pill instead, there are various herbal pills that include the above-listed herbs and others.

Animal wisdom. Cats and dogs seek out and eat couch grass when they have bladder problems. Couch grass has a high concentration of mucilage, which has a soothing effect on mucous membranes. Take one teaspoon of the root and simmer it for 30 minutes in 1½ pints of water. Drink cold, one swallow or one tablespoon at a time.

Spanish fly? Olé! Spanish fly, commonly called by its Latin name *Cantharis* by those involved with homeopathic medicine, is very effective for certain types of bladder infections. If you have a great deal of burning during and after urination, a frequent desire to urinate, and tend to pass urine only in drops, *Cantharis* 6 or 30, taken every four hours, should be tried. If it doesn't work within 48 hours, it wasn't the correct medicine, and you can stop taking it. A different homeopathic medicine to consider is *Aconite* 6 or 30 (monkshood), which is good for those bladder infections triggered by being chilled and which had a sudden onset. When the bladder infection seems to be triggered by sexual intercourse, sexual abuse, or an experience of humiliation, try *Staphysagria* 30 (staveacre).

*A **silver lining.*** Colloidal silver seems to have natural antiseptic properties that can fight infection. It is commonly available in health food stores.

Clean up your act ... carefully. Some women are sensitive to certain soaps, laundry detergents, bubble baths, contraceptive jellies, and dyes. Avoid feminine hygiene sprays, packaged douches, and scented toilet paper. Stick to natural, toxin-free products, and avoid these potential irritants.

Speaking of emptying yourself. Are you pissed off and holding it in? Are you afraid to let go? Your body may be giving you a message. Remember, anyone can get angry, but to get mad at the right person, at the right time, and in the right way is most therapeutic.

Watch what you mix with antibiotics. Research has now shown that grapefruit juice and certain mineral supplements (calcium, magnesium, and zinc) can inactivate certain antibiotics. You may need to choose one or the other.

7

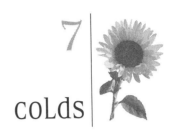

coLds

"Don't fight forces; use them."
—BUCKMINSTER FULLER

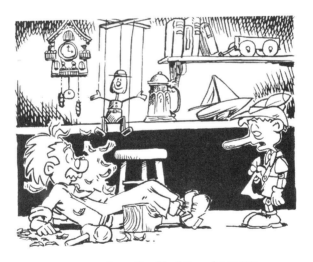

I'm sorry, Gepetto. Next time I sneeze,
I'll use super-strength tissues.

Have you ever wondered what that stuff coming out of your nose is when you have a cold? It's amazing how many smart people don't know the answer to this question and how few people (smart or otherwise) are interested in knowing. Well, it's important to know what it is because this knowledge will actually help you to cure it.

The common cold is the result of a viral infection, and the mucus is a liquid vehicle that eliminates the dead viruses and the body's dead white blood cells that have valiantly fought the viruses. The nasal discharge that you experience with a cold is, thus, a healthy response to an infection.

Now that you know that this gooey-gluey stuff out of your nose is the body performing an important healing function, you can understand that treating it with a clothes-pin as a way to stop the discharge doesn't make sense. And yet, many people take over-the-counter cold drugs that do about as much good. These drugs dry up the mucus that the body creates in its effort to flush dead viruses and white blood cells out of the body. It is no wonder that such drugs only work temporarily and cause various side effects, including congestion and drowsiness.

Scientists have identified more than 200 different viruses that cause the common cold, and more are being discovered all the time. Despite modern medical advances, physicians and drug companies remain stymied on how to effectively prevent or treat this all-too-common affliction. Perhaps a primary reason is our own inadequate medical model that seeks to attack and suppress symptoms rather than stimulate and augment the body's inherent healing efforts.

The common cold lasts anywhere from a couple of days to a couple of weeks. Infants and children usually suffer from six colds a year, teenagers usually get three or four colds a year, and the number of colds that adults get tends to decline throughout their life, except for those who are exposed to children who have colds.

It is generally assumed that adults who get more than a couple colds a year may have a weak immune system. On the other hand, some people who have a very weak immune system may be so sick that they cannot muster enough defensive reaction to create inflammatory symptoms of a common cold. Such is the paradox of health: Just because you don't get sick doesn't mean that you're healthy.

Because the nasal discharge from a cold is a healthy defensive reaction of the body, it has been said, "Don't cure a cold; let a cold cure you." If, however, you want to augment and speed up the body's efforts to heal itself, consider these strategies. If you are experiencing other symptoms, too, check out the appropriate chapters in this book for additional methods.

Is it starve a cold and feed a fever? Or, is it feed a cold and starve a fever? Neither! It is probably better to simply eat when you're hungry, and not eat when you're not. Just make sure to get plenty of fluids, especially water, broth, juices, and herb teas.

Supplement yourself. Take one gram of vitamin C every two hours, zinc gluconate lozenges every two hours, and 25,000 IU of vitamin A per day. Reduce your vitamin C dose if diarrhea develops (this is a sign that you've taken too much).

Seek out fresh air. Because a cold impairs your breathing, it is important go outside or keep windows in your house open (at least a little) in order to get fresh air and optimize respiration.

Take a sauna. Sweat it out, and it (the virus) may come out in the wash.

Don't get it handed to you. You are actually more likely to catch a cold from shaking the hand of a cold sufferer than kissing him or her. Cold sufferers shed their cold viruses onto their hands, then spread it to other people's hands, which eventually touch their nose or mouth and infect themselves. Perhaps even more dangerous is nose-to-nose Eskimo kissing, even though it may be therapeutic to the cold sufferer.

Let lemons squeeze the cold out of you. Lemons not only have vitamin C in them; they also have what one grandmother calls "natural corrosive action on mucus buildup" (one grandmother with a rather technical vocabulary, that is). Make some lemonade with equal parts of fresh lemon juice and water, and add a pinch of cayenne pepper and some honey (not too much, though). This drink will work better when it is tart and hot, but avoid boiling the lemon juice because it will significantly reduce its vitamin C content. It is best to just heat the water. Cayenne is known to help stimulate mucous membranes, loosen mucus, and increase circulation. Gargle with the first couple of gulps, and then drink the rest.

Herbal brews to bruise a cold. There are numerous herb teas that can help the body heal a cold. Brew one or more of the following herbs to make a tea: ginger (one ounce per pint of water), hyssop (one ounce/pint), peppermint (½-ounce/pint), rosehips (½-ounce/pint), and sage (¼-ounce/pint).

An herbal immune stimulant. Echinacea (purple coneflower) is one of the powerful herbs that can stimulate the

immune system, enabling it to more effectively fight a cold.
At the first sign of a sniffle, cough, or sneeze, take a dropperful (30 drops) of the echinacea extract. Take it once a day
for three or four days. Please note that liquid extracts or
tinctures tend to be considerably more effective than capsules of this herb (even though capsules are cheaper).
Instead, you might consider taking extracts of echinacea
and goldenseal together, but please know that goldenseal
is quite bitter (it really tastes like medicine!). Although
echinacea is a useful herb to fight a cold once you have
begun to develop symptoms, there is inadequate evidence
at present for its ability to prevent colds before any symptoms develop.

Steam it out. Eucalyptus and tea tree oil are powerful natural antiseptics. One or two drops of eucalyptus or tea
tree oil in a bowl of hot water can clear out your head
quite rapidly. Put a towel over your head and inhale the
steam.

Garlic keeps the evil cold spirits away. Whether it's
because garlic scares cold viruses or because the enzymes
within it devour the viruses, garlic can prevent the development of a cold. It is most effective if taken during the
early stages of infection. Consider eating two to four peeled
raw cloves, although you probably should only consider
this if you're living or working with people who love and

appreciate you! Consider chewing some fresh parsley afterwards; it's a natural breath freshener. If you want to be around others or you can't handle chewing on garlic cloves, there are now odorless garlic capsules available that are equally effective. Take two capsules three times a day.

The old standby: a bowl of Mama's hot chicken soup. Eat it as often as you think your mother would recommend it. It really works!

Homeopathic vitamin C. A homeopathic medicine to consider is *Aconitum* 6 or 30 if your symptoms include a rapid onset of a cold after exposure to cold weather or a cold, dry wind. Fever, restlessness, great thirst, and even a sense of anxiety may accompany the cold symptoms. *Aconitum* is only effective if you use it within the first 24 hours after the onset of symptoms. Take it every four hours. You won't need to take it for more than 24 hours. If you feel better after just one or two doses, stop there; you won't need any more.

No tears for onions. We all know that cutting onions causes watery eyes and a runny nose. More precisely, the runny nose is a profuse, clear, watery and burning discharge that tends to irritate the nostrils. Because onions cause this pattern of symptoms, they also can help to cure it when given in homeopathic doses. Take *Allium cepa* 6 or 30 (made from onions) every four hours if your symptoms match this pattern. You won't need to take it for more than 24 hours, and stop taking it as soon as improvement occurs.

Plant yourself. Indoor plants provide valuable moisture to the air and reduce the dry atmosphere from centrally heated buildings, thus minimizing the drying effect on nasal passages and the throat.

Grow facial hair. Hair acts as a cold-virus filter when it's abundant around the nose and mouth. This isn't a one-minute form of healing, isn't appropriate for half of us, and isn't foolproof, but hey, any additional help in preventing colds is always welcome!

When feet run, your nose won't. Research has shown that exercise at least temporarily stimulates white blood cells, thus fending off cold viruses. If, however, you're feeling achy or fatigued, don't exercise.

Drown your troubles in the ocean. If you live near salt water and swimming in it does not chill you too much, go for a dip. Swimming in salt water stimulates your nose to drain ... and drain ... and drain. The only problem with this strategy is that if everyone did it, the ocean would be less salty and a lot more ... yucky.

8

constipation

"There is no disease but stagnation,
no remedy but circulation."
—CHINESE PROVERB

When you consider that your large intestine is approximately 5 feet long, and your small intestine is 20 feet long, it's amazing that anything finds its way out of your body at all.

So many people in Western civilization experience constipation that many doctors dismiss it and consider it unworthy of their attention. Although constipation itself is not an illness, it is a symptom of something wrong. Is your diet adequate? Is there too much stress in your life? Were you exposed to certain toxic substances? Is it a side effect from a medication? Even though constipation won't kill you, it can lead to a general state of lowered health, for sluggish stools lead to sluggish people, physically and mentally.

Constipation itself is not a disease, but it can certainly *lead* to disease. Of particular concern is that it can lead to bad breath, body odor, and hemorrhoids. If that ain't scary, how about the fact that it can cause varicose veins, headaches, and insomnia. Well, okay, if you really want to be scared, you should know that it can also lead to depression, diverticulitis (it even sounds painful), and bowel cancer.

We all know what defecated matter smells like. Well, imagine that stuff sitting inside you longer than it should be. It is surprising that constipation isn't considered a disease, and how come there aren't any nonprofit organizations, such as the Foundation for Constipation Relief, trying to raise money and consciousness about the problems that people suffer as a result of constipation? I guess we know why there aren't any such organizations. Who would want to be its spokesperson? Who would want to admit that they are members? What slogans could be used that wouldn't be offensive or humorous?

The most common cause of constipation is our processed, low-fiber, high-fat and high-sugar diet. Food companies have, for better or worse, come to the aid of people with constipation and are adding fiber to everything. Ironically, in order to create white bread, food companies commonly denature the whole wheat grain and then add fiber back into the bread. Some food companies add "powdered cellulose" to their bread recipes. Although this certainly adds fiber to the diet, powdered cellulose, also known as sawdust, isn't the ideal way to get your fiber.

Older people are five times more likely to suffer from constipation than younger people are. While this may be partly due to poor diet, inadequate fluid consumption, or lack of exercise, it is also because of past laxative use. Millions of people today, especially older folks, are addicted to laxatives. Although these drugs provide temporary relief, they do nothing to remedy the *cause* of the constipation. Worse yet, whenever you get something done for you easily, you're not able to do it for yourself as well, leading to chronic constipation problems.

Most people don't realize that coffee has strong laxative properties. People sometimes become addicted to it, not simply for the taste or the caffeine, but because of coffee's effects on their bowels. People who sharply reduce their coffee intake tend to become constipated temporarily. However, there are safer ways to regulate your bowels than drinking coffee.

Here are some strategies that you can use for yourself. They will be helpful in navigating the 25 feet or more of intestines so that whatever you put into your body will be able to easily find its way out.

Do, but don't overdo, fiber! The best sources of fiber are grains, legumes, and fresh fruits and vegetables. Whole wheat bread and brown rice are naturally preferred over white bread and white rice. Bran, prunes, and apples are particularly good sources of fiber; however, be aware that increasing fiber intake too rapidly or simply eating too much of it can cause indigestion, gas, and diarrhea.

Lubricate yourself. Drink six to eight glasses of water a day.

Bulk up. Take a "bulk former," such as psyllium preparations, available from herb stores or in commercial form from pharmacies. (Try Metamucil or Konsyl—the latter is preferred because it does not contain sugar or Nutrasweet.) Flaxseed and linseed are other good sources of bulk. At least once a day, grind the flaxseed or linseed in a coffee grinder; and add it to a cup of water, juice, broth, or cereal.

Olive oil and lemon. Take one tablespoon of olive oil and the juice of one lemon just before bedtime and upon rising in the morning (don't eat any food for at least 30 minutes afterwards). Commonly called "a liver flush," this combination is thought to stimulate liver function and improve overall digestion and elimination of food. Another effective strategy is to mix one lemon with one cup of warm water and drink it before bedtime and upon getting up in the morning.

Massage your abdomen from the outside and the inside. Massage your abdomen from the outside in a kneading type of motion. Massaging your abdomen from the inside is another useful exercise: Bend halfway over, placing your hands on your mid-thighs, exhale completely, and then empty your abdomen further by pumping your abdominal muscles up and down; try to do six pumps per breath. The more advanced internal massage is one in which the right side of the abdomen is pumped first, and then the left side is pumped next in the same breath.

Avoid laxatives, unless you want short-term relief and long-term constipation. If you feel you must take a laxative, take an herbal laxative, although the body can become reliant on herbal laxatives, too. Senna and cascara bark are probably the best. One way to take senna is to place a teaspoon of senna leaves in boiling water and let steep for 30 minutes. Drink ½ cup in the morning and ½ cup in the evening. As for cascara bark, take one tablespoon in capsule form before bedtime.

Herbal stool softeners. Aloe vera, either fresh or in juice form, can help soften stools and make them easier to eliminate. Figure out for yourself what dose and which frequency of dose works best for you, and please know that in treating constipation with herbs, it is best not to take them for more than three consecutive weeks. Give your own body a chance to do things on its own, too.

Supplements to consider. Acidophilus provides friendly bacteria to help improve digestion and elimination. Apple pectin gives useful fiber. Vitamin C in high doses (5–0 grams per day) can loosen stools. Alfalfa or chlorophyll can help detoxify the body.

Avoid the drug plugs. If you are taking any medications, check to see if they promote constipation. Painkillers and antidepressants are two common types of drugs that usually *cause* constipation. Over-the-counter antacids that contain aluminum can also constipate.

Avoid the food and vitamin plugs, too. Certain foods such as milk, cheese, and white flour products; and certain vitamins such as iron and calcium supplements can cause constipation.

Exercise! If your body is lazy, you can expect your stools to be lazy, too.

Bounce in a squatting position. Flexing anal muscles by squatting and bouncing helps build up anal muscle tone.

Create a ritual. It is sometimes useful to sit on the toilet at the same time every day, even if you don't feel the urge to defecate. It is generally best to do this either in the morning or after some exercise.

Get in touch with your inner plumber. When your intestines are not pushing things along as they should, perhaps a visualization exercise that simulates Roto-rooter action moving thing down the drain will help. This strategy may not be adequate if used without other methods. Just like the Islamic saying, "Trust in God, but tie your camel to a palm tree," you should trust your inner plumber, but keep eating your fiber!

9

coughs

"A cough is something that you yourself can't help, but everybody else does on purpose just to torment you."
—OGDEN NASH

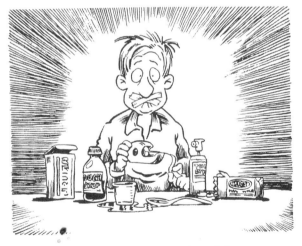

Another unproven treatment for
the common cough.

A cough can expel air at a velocity of up to 500 miles per hour. Such is the power of the body in its efforts to rid the respiratory system of irritants and toxins. It is no wonder that people feel uncomfortable in a theater when sitting immediately in front of a person with a cough.

The common cough is an effective primary defense of the human organism. It is therefore surprising that some over-the-counter drugs pride themselves on being "cough suppressants." Besides being a questionably effective strategy in curing a cough, such drugs can delay proper diagnosis of a serious illness such as lung cancer, emphysema, poisoning, or pneumonia.

The cough itself is not a disease; it is a symptom of a disease. Like other efforts that primarily try to control or suppress an individual symptom, drug treatments do not necessarily treat the underlying disease. A more healing therapy would be something that aids the body's efforts to clear respiratory obstruction or irritation.

There are innumerable types of coughs. There are dry and wet coughs, hacking and barking coughs, deep and shallow coughs, and single and rapid-fire coughs. Individualizing treatment is important, but difficult. Basically, dry coughs should be treated first with humidification strategies and lozenges, while wet coughs can benefit from natural expectorants. As for the various other types of coughs, experiment with different strategies, and don't forget to breathe. The following methods point you in this direction in a way that won't take your breath away.

Take an expectoration cocktail. If you have a wet cough with mucus that obstructs your breathing, mix the juice of a lemon, one tablespoon of honey, and ¼ teaspoon of cayenne pepper in warm water. The astringency and the acidity of the lemon cause the tissues to contract and help to dissolve and dislodge mucus. The honey soothes the mucous membranes and respiratory tract, and the cayenne pepper adds power to the body's ability to expectorate. Gargle with this cocktail, and then swallow it. Take it as needed. Hardy individuals might consider adding crushed garlic and/or crushed fresh ginger, but please know that all forms of this combination of ingredients are not what anyone might call tasty.

An expectoration cocktail for the brave. The onion is a great mucus dissolver. Blend or juice an onion, and add honey to it. Take a couple of tablespoons of this mixture as needed.

Other natural expectorants. Garlic! Eat a clove of it if you're brave and not planning to entertain (the less fainthearted or the more sociable types can take the odorless garlic capsules). An easier strategy is making sage tea and adding garlic to it. Another herbal method is to mix elecampane and mullein. Elecampane is an herb that contains helenin, a powerful antiseptic and bactericidal alkaloid. Elecampane helps to expectorate the mucus, and mullein is soothing to the respiratory tract. For children, consider using wild cherry bark tea.

Treat your cough gingerly. Chew on a piece of ginger root, and swallow the juice. Ginger has both anti-inflammatory and antioxidant agents that help to heal lung tissue and help break up mucus congestion.

Herbal lozenges. White horehound is another herbal expectorant. White horehound lozenges are commonly sold in drugstores and health food stores.

Vaporize yourself. Inhale steam from a vaporizer, or put a towel over your head and stand over the steam rising from a pot of boiling water. Consider adding a couple of drops of the herb hyssop to the water, and breathe this steamy air for five to ten minutes. Hyssop has been used since ancient times for its antiseptic and emollient (soothing) properties. Penicillin mold is known to thrive on its leaves.

Fire and ice treatment. Alternate hot and cold water in the shower, every three minutes or so. Make certain to let the water hit your chest and back.

Avoid milk products. The lactose in milk is a complex sugar that is difficult to digest for some (not all!) people. It can encourage more mucus production in people who have a difficult time digesting it, and this can further congest breathing.

Spit it out. If and when you are able to hack up phlegm, don't swallow it—spit it out. Your body has successfully disengaged this mucus from your breathing passageways with the intent of getting rid of it. If you are worried about what Ms. Manners might be thinking, daintily spit it into a napkin or find a nearby wastebasket.

Where there's smoke, there's fire. Avoid first- and secondhand smoke. This irritant can exacerbate your breathing difficulties. If you have a cough and you're still smoking, remember that cancer cures smoking, permanently. Try another cure.

Supplement your breathing. Vitamin C can help heal your cough if it is the result of a viral or bacterial infection. Take 1,000 mg of vitamin C three times a day. Vitamin E can prevent and treat the cellular damage from cigarette smoke, dust, soot, pollen, smog, or other airborne pollutants. Take 400 IU of vitamin E twice a day.

Channel your mother. She is telling you to stand up

straight so that you can take a full breath. She is also telling you not to wear clothing so tight that it inhibits your breathing. Now that you're thinking about your posture, do some exercises that will help it, such as stretching exercises that roll your shoulders back. This exercise can help you breathe more easily, which is important whether you have a cough or not.

Relax your shoulders. Too often people walk around all day with tense shoulders. Shoulders should not normally be at or near ear height; when you wear your shoulder as earrings, it is considerably more difficult to take a healthy deep breath. One good exercise to relax the shoulders is to lift them to your ears and tighten them . . . then relax them.

Get loose. A cough tends to tighten your chest and back muscles, which then makes it more difficult to take a full breath. Do some yoga exercises that help to loosen you up a bit. Do the cobra: Lie on your abdomen with your palms lying flat under your shoulders. Lift your torso off the ground using your hands and arms, while keeping your head up and back. Take several breaths in this raised position, and then slowly return to lying flat. Rest, then repeat this exercise several times. After this, do some back rolls: Lie on your back with your hands wrapped around knees that are bent and as close to your chest as feels comfortable. Gently rock forward and backward.

Chant your way to health. Unless talking causes a coughing attack, try sitting in a relaxing position and uttering a single sound. It can be "ahhhhhh," "ommmmmm," "yummmmmm," or whatever feels good to you. Such sounds can be soothing and can help to relax you so that the respiratory mucus falls into your digestive tract.

Keep the third lung healthy. Not only does the skin cover you, it also breathes for you. During respiratory problems, the skin often becomes drier. Do not smear oily creams over it that plug up the pores and make it difficult for this third lung to function. It's helpful to stimulate the skin with a loofah brush.

Re-spirit yourself. The very word *respiratory* contains the concept of "re-spirit." Are your spirits down? Have you noticed that you tend to breathe more shallowly whenever you're depressed? Such breathing invites a cough. Re-spirit yourself (see the section on Depression), and you'll find you'll take deeper breaths, and your cough will spirit itself away.

10

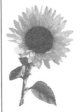

Depression

"Depression is melancholy minus its charm."
—SUSAN SONTAG

D epression lowers the spirits and drowns the eyes in sorrow, although tears aren't the only reason why depressed people sometimes can't see straight. Depression also caves in the chest, slumps the shoulders, and inhibits full breathing, usually forcing unhappy people to try to catch their breath by frequently sighing. It is sometimes said that depression brings you down to sighs (my apology to those readers who get depressed from bad puns).

Depression certainly has more than physical effects. Its real ravages are psychological and spiritual. It creates a serious case of blah-itis, which is an inflamed state of the blahs. People with the blahs lose interest in the things they usually love and begin really hating things that they normally feel so-so about. They tend to doubt themselves, others, and in fact, they doubt just about everything—except their own doubts. In more serious cases, they may wonder if life is meaningful or worthwhile, and in the most extreme cases, they stop reading self-help books that try to make them laugh. This is when depression can be seriously depressing.

A major trauma can certainly be the straw that breaks that poor old camel's back, or you may get pushed over the edge by an accumulation of small stresses. Some people feel depressed during normally "good times," such as the holidays; and some women experience the "baby blues" shortly after giving birth. Every phase of life has its own potential for stress and depression.

Viral or bacterial infection, organic disease, or hormonal disorders also can precipitate depression. It can be drug induced, especially as a result of taking barbiturates, amphetamines, birth control pills, and alcohol. It can stem from exposure to certain environmental poisons, and sometimes it seems that depression can even be contagious— one person's depressed condition can certainly bring others down, too.

With all these possible triggers floating around, it is no wonder that virtually everybody experiences some depression at least one time in their life. There is no reason to feel guilty about an occasional bout of depression, unless, of course, you're trying hard to meet your annual guilt quota.

The common classifications of depression are unipolar, bipolar, major, and psychotic. Unipolar refers to depression without manic highs (oh no!). Bipolar refers to alternating depressive states and manic high episodes (oh no, oh yes!). Psychotic refers to depression along with hallucinations and/or delusions (the good news here is that it is usually in color!). And major depression is characterized by the inability to be cheered up (no color at all!).

In every dark and depressive period in one's life, there is also some light somewhere. Getting in touch with that light is important, but this is not always easy to do. It seems as though everyone has his or her own ideas about moving out of the depressed state of mind. Understanding the various theories about depression may be helpful in treating it, but as psychiatrist Carl Jung once said, "Learn your theories as well as you can, but put them aside when you touch the miracle of a living soul."

Whether you fully understand the reasons for your depression or not, here are some sensible strategies for reconnecting with and spreading your light. Albert Camus, well-known writer on existentialism and loneliness, once wrote, "In the depth of winter, I finally learned that there was in me an invincible summer."

Exercise those demons out of you! Exercise is not only helpful for building a fit body, but it also helps to create a sound mind. Getting your body moving seems to help keep your mind out of the depths of depression. Exercise that involve the long muscles, such as jogging, swimming, and bicycling; and playing basketball, football, or tennis, are the most beneficial.

St. John can help. Solid research has shown that St. John's wort *(Hypericum perforatum)* is as effective as, and considerably safer than, conventional antidepressive drugs in treating a wide range of people suffering from mild to moderately severe depression. Rather than making a tea of this herb, it is best to take it in pill or liquid extract form. It is generally recommended to take 2–4 g of the herb, or 0.4-2.7 mg of total hypericin (one of its active ingredients) with a standardized hyperforin content. If you are already taking a conventional antidepressant drug, you should know that taking St. John's wort along with it may lead to an overabundance of serotonin, which can result in agitation, sweating, lightheadedness, and headaches.

Supplement and feed your mood. A B-complex vitamin and the amino acid tryptophan help increase the brain's release of serotonin, which is a natural antidepressant. Foods that are high in tryptophan are complex carbohydrates (found in potatoes, pasta, grains, and garbanzo beans), but consider avoiding wheat, because wheat gluten is sometimes linked to depressive states. Foods that are high in serotonin include bananas, soybeans, nuts, turkey, and tuna.

Don't overdo protein. Too much protein can inhibit the brain's uptake of tryptophan and increase feelings of depression.

Don't forget to breathe. It is common for depressed people to breathe shallowly, which tends to create a physical depression to go with the psychological depression. You can help get out of this depressed state by taking full, deep breaths more often. Alternate nostril breathing creates a rhythmic profusion of air, which further enhances oxygenation of the body. To do this type of breathing, sit comfortably with your back straight, exhale fully, close the right nostril with your right thumb, and inhale slowly through your left nostril. After you have inhaled fully through your left nostril, close it with your right ring finger, and exhale through your right nostril. Keep your left nostril closed, and inhale through your right nostril. Then hold the right nostril closed, and exhale through your left nostril. Repeat this process for a couple of minutes.

Befriend a friend. When you are depressed, you tend to keep to yourself and wallow in your own misery. Don't suffer alone—extend yourself, and talk to or visit a friend.

Help someone else. Being with, talking to, and helping others less fortunate will not only take your mind off your depression, it will help make you feel better about yourself and your own life.

Befriend a pet. Adopting a pet cat, dog, frog, or tarantula—or whatever—is wonderfully therapeutic. You will have a friend to talk to who will listen to your every word and provide you with unconditional love—and a pet is less expensive than a therapist.

Give yourself credit for something, anything. When you are depressed, you tend to blame yourself for everything and rarely acknowledge anything good about yourself or your life. Look for what is going right. By shining a little light onto this positive side, perhaps you will find that glimmer of sunshine peeking out from behind the clouds.

Swear off sin. Alcohol, cigarettes, drugs (recreational and therapeutic), caffeine, sugar, and junk food can all depress you, physically and psychologically. Perhaps your depression is telling you that what you are doing to your body is bringing you down.

Join the coffee generation. Coffee, like sugar, can lead to various problems, but small amounts can also be beneficial for some people, especially during bouts of depression. Caffeine molecules have been shown to displace certain neurotransmitters and help to keep the "good mood" chemicals in circulation. Coffee is fast-acting, and the effects can last three to six hours. Despite these benefits, be aware that coffee is like a drug and has side effects, including anxiety and panic disorders. Also, withdrawal from consistently large amounts of coffee can lead to depressive states. Because of these various problems, safer methods should be considered before resorting to this strategy. Don't drink more than one cup a day during times of depression.

Let there be light. Light has been found to affect brain chemicals in a way that reduces depressive states. If it is dark and gloomy outside for a prolonged period and if it isn't possible to travel to a sunnier place, try lifting the shades in your home, opening windows, turning on brighter lights, and wearing lighter and brighter clothing.

Get out of here. Consider "travel therapy." Changing your routine, going on a vacation, and adding a little adventure to your life is often therapeutic.

Write on! Keeping a journal of your thoughts, feelings, and experiences provides a wonderful and often helpful catharsis. Writing can also help you come to a better understanding of your depression, which may help lift its veil so that you can better understand and appreciate yourself and your experience.

Draw it out of you. Draw or paint what you are feeling. Not only will it feel good to do so, but you may even get a valuable work of art out of it.

Let it rain! If the tears are there, cry! Don't bottle up your feelings. Tears contain chemicals that need to be released.

Flowers can help. Yes, flowers often make a person feel appreciated, but in addition to giving or getting flowers, they can also be used therapeutically. The Bach Flower Remedies are 38 flowers that British physician Edward Bach discovered as being beneficial for various emotional states. Dr. Bach found Sweet Chestnut, Mustard, and Crab Apple to be most useful for treating depression. These flower products are often available at health food stores.

Pamper yourself. Give yourself time to appreciate yourself and your life. Take a hot bath. Relax in a comfortable place. Listen to beautiful music. Take a walk in nature or anyplace that feels good to you. Get a massage. Read a good uplifting book. Reread *this* book!

11

diarrhea

"Whatever is produced in haste goes hastily to waste."
—SA'DI, GULISTAN (1258)

Diarrhea is, loosely speaking (hardy-har-har), the passage of too-frequent and too-soft stools. Diarrhea occurs when the fluid contents of the small intestine are so rapidly hurried through the large intestines that fluid is not adequately absorbed and is then discharged. This elimination catches some people off-guard and with their pants down, so to speak.

Like vomiting, diarrhea is a defense mechanism that the body deploys in order to rapidly discharge germs, toxins, and irritants. Bacteria actually make up approximately 10 percent of the bulk of normal stools; this percentage increases if a person's diarrhea is a result of eating bacteria-contaminated foods or drinks. Because of this high bacteria content, drugs that attempt to constipate a person who has diarrhea can be harmful because they reduce his or her ability to discharge potentially dangerous germs. Often, it is best to let diarrhea "run" its course.

Diarrhea should not always be left untreated, however. Sometimes diarrhea is symptomatic of a more serious disorder such as ulcerative colitis, which may require medical attention. If the diarrhea lasts more than two days or if the stools are either bloody or look like black tar, seek medical attention. Also, diarrhea can create its own problems, as with an infant whose diarrhea leads to dehydration. Still, the vast majority of people who experience diarrhea should not try to suppress this symptom immediately. Instead, here are some simple strategies that can help the body resolve this itself.

Do the Zen diet. Eat nothing. This resting of your digestive system often helps to reestablish a healthy bowel. Fasting also helps by not getting in the way of what your body, in its infinite wisdom, is trying to expel.

Water yourself. Diarrhea leads to greater excretion of bodily fluids, so it is important to replace them by drinking plenty of water. Persistent or acute diarrhea may also excrete important nutrients from the body. Since solid food is sometimes difficult to digest during bouts of diarrhea, drink diluted fruit juice with a pinch of salt, and alternate drinking it with a glass of carbonated water that contains ¼ teaspoon baking soda. Drink one cup after each bout of diarrhea.

It's barbecue time, sort of. Take activated charcoal. This product is commonly sold in pharmacies and health food stores and has been found to stifle bacterial growth. Take four tablets every hour until the diarrhea subsides. If the diarrhea persists after a couple of days, consider other strategies.

A pinch here and a pinch there. Put a pinch of cinnamon and a pinch of cayenne pepper in two cups of boiling water, and let it simmer for 20 minutes. Take two tablespoons every hour.

Be good to your bowels, and they won't run out on you. Slippery elm bark is a tried-and-true herbal remedy for diarrhea. It is both nourishing and soothing to the bowels. Add one ounce of slippery elm bark to one quart of boiling water, and let it simmer until approximately one pint remains. Add honey, if necessary, to soothe the palate, and take one teaspoon every 30 minutes.

A golden seal to help plug up the runs. The herb goldenseal contains an alkaloid called berberine, which has been shown to help treat acute diarrhea caused by certain bacteria. It is also helpful in preventing diarrhea in those people traveling in underdeveloped countries. Consider taking it one week prior to going away, during your trip, and one week after returning home. Take the tincture

(1–1½ teaspoons), fluid extract (¼–½ teaspoon), or powdered solid extract (250–500 mg) three times a day.

Acupinch yourself. Pinch or press one, two, or all of the following acupressure points: Spleen 16 is below the edge of the rib cage a half inch inside from the nipple line; Stomach 36 is four finger widths below the kneecap and one finger width to the outside of the shinbone; Conception Vessel 6 is two finger widths immediately below the belly button; Spleen 4 is at the juncture of the big and the second toes. If a spot feels a bit tender, you've found it. Press it for at least ten seconds, release, and then repeat a couple more times.

Eat the BRATY bunch. If you have an appetite, eat foods from the **BRATY** bunch: **b**ananas, (white) **r**ice, **a**pplesauce, **t**oast, and **y**ogurt (not necessarily together). These foods are relatively easy to digest for most people, and they're nourishing.

Get cultured. Miso soup and yogurt are known to contain a rich amount of *Lactobacillus acidophilus* bacteria that is useful for digesting foods. In addition to eating these foods, consider purchasing acidophilus supplements at a health food store.

Kelp yourself. Kelp (a type of seaweed that is available in pill form) can help replace lost minerals. You might want to add some potassium, too, because this important mineral is also lost when you have diarrhea.

Run to garlic. If you are diagnosed with parasites, eat lots of raw or capsulated garlic. Parasites must not be Italian, because they hate garlic!

Arsenic but not old lace. A homeopathic dose of arsenic (called *Arsenicum*) is an effective medicine for diarrhea from food poisoning. It is also often effective for diarrhea when the sick person has what are considered "*Arsenicum* symptoms": great thirst, but for only sips at a time; restlessness combined with weakness, a chill with possibly a fever, and a worsening of symptoms around midnight. If your symptoms match many of these, take *Arsenicum* 12 or 30 every four hours for one or two days.

Be anti-antacid and anti-antibiotic. Certain drugs induce diarrhea as a side effect. Antacids have an ingredient in them that causes diarrhea, and antibiotics kill the beneficial bacteria, making it more difficult to absorb nutrients in the bowel.

Don't drink just anything. Coffee, black tea, and alcohol can lead to diarrhea.

Every body does not need milk. The American milk industry has tried to tell us that "every body needs milk," and the British milk industry has tried to make the British believe that "every body needs bottle" (*bottle* is British slang for "machismo"). These industrialized public relations efforts are messing with our minds ... and our bowels. Approximately 80 percent of black Americans and between 5 and 15 percent of white Americans are lactose intolerant. Milk is not good for every body, unless you consider running to the toilet to be a good aerobic exercise.

Certain sugars aren't so sweet. Fructose and sorbitol (in sugarless gums and candies) can cause diarrhea. Avoid them if you have the tendency to run.

Avoid too much of a good thing. Fiber is good for preventing constipation, but too many fiber-rich foods, such as prunes, figs, beans, and bran, can loosen you more than you may want.

Changing religions isn't helpful. Crohn's disease, a chronic diarrheal condition, is more often experienced by Jewish people than any other group. Unfortunately, converting to another religion will not be a very effective treatment.

Are you hurrying yourself and your bowels? Do you talk fast, walk fast, eat fast, and drive fast? Are you not finishing what you begin? Do you have a tendency to want to get something over with as soon as possible? Are you restlessly and chronically running away from something? If you're not fully digesting your life and want to move on to the next thing before you're finished doing what you're doing, you can expect your bowels to act in the same way. Take your time in life. Don't hurry. Enjoy what's happening in the moment. Affirm to yourself: *I fully enjoy doing things slowly.*

Anticipation is as strong as any bacteria. Anticipation can cause diarrhea just as effectively as bacteria can. Worries, anxieties, and other anticipatory emotional states can make your bowels feel insecure, too. Repeat to yourself: *I am at peace with myself, and I appreciate where I am right now.*

12

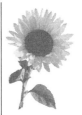

earaches

"The reason why we have two ears and only one mouth
is that we may listen the more and talk the less."
—ZENO OF CITIUM (300 B.C.)

Earaches are caused by various factors, including bacterial or viral infections, allergies, swimming, or changes in altitude due to flying or mountain climbing. Most commonly, earaches result when the Eustachian tube, which connects the middle ear to the cavity behind the nose, is blocked, causing the trapped fluids to become a perfect breeding ground for bacterial or viral infection.

Doctors usually prescribe antibiotics for ear infections; however, these drugs do not always work, and what's worse is that some research suggests that there is an increased probability of experiencing another ear infection when antibiotics are used. Sadly, too many doctors overprescribe antibiotics for earaches. Perhaps the medical community has its collective Eustachian tube blocked so that it cannot hear and respond to research on the limitations of these drugs. When you consider that many earaches are caused by viral infections or allergies for which antibiotics are useless, it makes sense to seek out alternative treatment.

Because the Eustachian tube in infants and children is very short, they are more prone than adults to ear infection. In fact, earaches are the number-one reason that parents take their child to a doctor. Infants who are taken to doctors for their regular checkups are occasionally diagnosed with an ear infection as a result of a reddened ear, and even though the infant is not noticeably ill or irritated, the child is prescribed antibiotics. However, because of the growing recognition that antibiotics are overprescribed for ear infections and because research has not adequately proven their efficacy, safer alternative treatments should be considered.

Earaches may be painful to the child, but they are frightening to parents. Parents who are unfamiliar with some simple home remedies inevitably feel helpless as they hear their child cry for help and yet can do nothing. In such instances, parents tend to feel more anxiety than the children feel pain. When the child gets recurrent ear infections, parents' fear of hearing loss adds to the anguish associated with this condition.

The following strategies are helpful for the little ears of children, as well as the ears of the rest of us.

Treat a cold and sore throat well. If a child's cold or sore throat worsens, it can lead to an ear infection. Read the section on Colds and Sore Throat so that you can help prevent ear problems.

Here's the rub. Massage the head, especially around the ears, though not the ears themselves. Massage whatever parts seem to feel sensitive to touch for at least one minute. You may want to massage them for another minute after a short rest.

Be fluid. Earaches sometimes result from mucus congestion in the nose and throat. Be certain to drink enough fluids. Warm liquids tend to be more soothing. However, avoid drinking milk, which can lead to more congestion.

Whether you're tired or not, yawn. Yawning helps to open the Eustachian tube, which can reduce ear pressure and help decrease fluid or pus buildup in the ear.

Chew your cud. Chewing and swallowing also helps to open the Eustachian tube, reduce ear pressure, and decrease ear pain. Research has even verified that chewing gum can help relieve earaches.

Steam it out. Steam inhalations or saunas may be helpful. These treatments create a pseudo-fever during which white blood cells become more active and can more effectively fight infection.

Use a liquid pillow. Wrap a towel around a hot water bottle, place it on the ear with the greatest amount of pain or redness, and use it like a pillow.

Avoid swimming. Being underwater can aggravate an ear infection.

Hunt for allergies. Some children are allergic to certain foods that weaken them and make them more susceptible to various illnesses, including ear infections. Perhaps the most common culprits are milk and other dairy foods. Every calf may need milk, but most humans don't. Consider using soy milk instead. Other common food allergies often stem from dairy products, wheat, eggs, citrus, corn, and peanut butter.

Let garlic get the demons out of those ears. Peel a clove of garlic, dip it in oil, and place it at the ear's opening (do not push it into the ear). Leave it there overnight unless it becomes too irritating.

Let's hear it for mullein oil! Place a couple of drops of mullein oil into the ear. Mullein is an herb, and many pharmacies and most herb stores sell the oil. If there is a discharge from the ear, it may signify that the eardrum is broken. Do not use any eardrops if this happens.

For those little infant ears. The tincture of *Plantago* (plantain) is an excellent remedy for infants who are experiencing teething at the same time they are having ear pains. This tincture should be diluted two parts of the remedy to one part water. Place a couple of drops in the ear, and rub some into the gum. This remedy is available at homeopathic pharmacies or herb stores.

Get cultured. Because many people with ear infections have often been given round after round of antibiotics, it is important to help the body reestablish the healthy bacteria in your intestines. Take an acidophilus supplement. The best strains are DDS and NCFM—if a supplement doesn't say that it includes these strains, then it doesn't.

It's as simple as ABC. There are three common homeopathic medicines for ear infection: *Aconitum* (monkshood), *Belladonna* (deadly nightshade), and *Chamomilla* (chamomile). *Aconitum* is usually given at the initial onset of ear symptoms, especially if it began after exposure to cold. *Belladonna* is given when a person with an ear infection has a noticeably reddened ear, ear canal, eardrum, and sometimes a flushed face. There is a sudden onset of symptoms, with pains that are throbbing, piercing, or shooting, sometimes extending to the throat. These pains are worse with motion and at night and usually have a fever concurrently. *Chamomilla* is indicated when people, usually infants, experience great pain and are extremely irritable because of it. They are impatient and cannot be consoled. They are very sensitive to touch, but are temporarily relieved by being rocked or carried. They may experience teething concurrent with their ear infection. Take the 6th or 30th potency every four hours for one or two days. Once improvement is experienced with a homeopathic medicine, it is no longer necessary to continue taking it.

Not just ABC! It isn't always as simply as ABC, because homeopathic doses of *Pulsatilla* (windflower) are often wonderfully effective in curing an ear infection. It is particularly useful for infants, children, and anyone who seeks sympathy and attention during an earache and who needs to be held. People who need this remedy tend to have the worst symptoms at night and when feeling warm. Such people like to have a window open for fresh air and for cool air. Even if they have a fever, they do not tend to be thirsty. Use the 6th or 30th potency every two hours if symptoms are intense, and every four to six hours if they are mild. Once improvement is experienced or if no significant improvement occurs in 48 hours, it is no longer necessary to take any more of this remedy.

An old-time and sure-fire cure. If you get an earache from getting water in your ear as a result of swimming or showering, put your head over to one side, pull the top of the ear upward and backward, and then squeeze a dropperful of equal parts white vinegar and rubbing alcohol into the ear. The alcohol absorbs the water, while the vinegar kills the bacteria or fungi that are growing in your soggy ear. Although this is an old-time cure, the American Academy of Otolaryngology (doctors who treat the ear, nose, and throat) now recommends it.

Give yourself a helping gland. Studies have shown that extracts from a calf's thymus gland can improve immune function, reduce childhood food allergies, and increase a child's resistance to chronic respiratory infections. Extracts from the thymus gland have, in particular, been beneficial to people with chronic middle ear infection. Consider taking 50 mg of thymus extract for each year of age of the earache sufferer (for example, a 12-year-old would receive 50 x 12 mg = 600 mg).

Breast-feeding is the best feeding. Breast-fed babies have been found to have fewer ear infections. Their immune systems seems better able to resist infection, and they are less prone to allergies and the ear infections that sometimes result from them.

Correct your bottle-feeding and breast-feeding techniques. Infants who tend to get ear infections should never be fed while they're lying flat. If they are, the milk has a tendency to go directly into the Eustachian tube and block it, leading to ear infections.

Don't take your earache lying down. Most earaches in both adults and children are aggravated by lying down because the Eustachian tubes are not draining. If you prop your head up while sleeping, or just sit up for a few minutes, you can sometimes ease the pain.

Avoid the smoke screen. There is a well-documented link between parental smoking and childhood ear infections. If you are a parent who smokes, stop—not just for your own sake—but for your child's. Also, do whatever you can to prevent your child from getting secondhand smoke from others.

Vacuum therapy. Tests have shown that rugs and carpets are approximately 20 times (!) dirtier than the average city sidewalk. An infant's or child's allergy leading to an earache can be set off by the dirt and dust in a rug, especially when the children spend much time crawling or playing on the floor. Vacuum frequently.

Pacify infants during air travel. Infants tend to experience great distress during air travel due to inadequate opening of the Eustachian tube from the rapid change in air pressure. To prevent this problem, infants should be nursed, given a pacifier, or placed on the bottle during takeoff and landing.

13

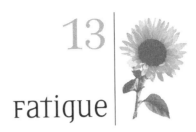

Fatigue

"Life is one long process of getting tired."
—SAMUEL BUTLER

Fatigue can make everything more difficult. Remote control for television is a godsend for the seriously fatigued, but unfortunately, there is no remote control for most of life's other activities.

Fatigue is a frustrating condition; not only does it affect one's physical energy, but it affects one's mental energy, too. Mental jogging becomes as difficult as physical jogging. Symptoms that commonly accompany fatigue include the inability to think clearly, sleep disturbances, constipation, apathy, depression, swollen glands, and difficulty reading.

Chronic fatigue syndrome has become one of the latest garbage-can diagnoses for various fatigue-related health problems. Some physicians think that it is caused by the Epstein-Barr virus; others think it's from the HBLV virus, and still others think that it's a mixture or "cocktail" of several viruses.

Some fatigue syndromes have nothing to do with viral infections, but could be the result of anemia, a thyroid problem, or some other disease. And some fatigue syndromes result from psychological problems, although in these cases, it is difficult to determine if the psychological problem caused the fatigue or vice versa.

Fatigue can be caused by overexertion, but it can also result from underexertion. An overstressed athlete is as likely to become as fatigued as a couch potato.

The fact that you've read this far means that you're not a total basket case. Here are some strategies to get you up, on your feet again, and raring to go.

Energy creates energy. Exercise may sound like an impossible dream when you're fatigued, but it does stimulate circulation and metabolism. Regular exercise usually enhances energy, but be careful not to exhaust yourself.

Take a cold shower. Taking a cold shower will really wake you up! If you're not brave enough to take one, then take a cold footbath, or simply splash your face with cold water.

Avoid cheap tricks. Drinking coffee and eating sweets may give you short-term energy, but they can lead to greater fatigue because these substances sap the adrenal glands and disrupt blood-sugar levels. Stay away from these energy robbers.

Go light on lunch. Large lunches, especially those with high-fat foods, commonly cause afternoon fatigue. Avoid them unless it's okay for you to sleep at your desk.

Watch your protein. Fatigue can result from having too much protein or too little. Make certain that you're getting enough but not too much. One meal per day, maybe two at the most, should have a food rich with protein. Meat and dairy products are sources of protein, but there are healthier alternatives. You can get complete protein meals with less fat by eating plenty of whole grains, vegetables, legumes, and seeds.

Start the day right. It is best to have a good breakfast. Whole-grain cereals—oatmeal, for example—have plenty of complex carbohydrates, which provide sustained energy.

Are your drugs putting you to sleep? Fatigue and tiredness are common side effects of various prescription and over-the-counter drugs. Sleeping pills may help you fall asleep, but they commonly lead to increased fatigue the next day. Other energy drainers are high blood pressure drugs, antihistamines, and cold and cough medicines.

Utilize your good times. Some people with fatigue find that they have more energy at specific times of the day or night. Make use of these times to do your more intensive tasks and to practice healing efforts.

Supplement your energy. Take vitamin C with meals three times a day; beta-carotene, B complex, and vitamin E twice a day; and a mixed mineral supplement once a day. Grapeseed extract is a powerful antioxidant—take it at least once a day. If you take these supplements with your meals, they usually will be easier to assimilate.

Herbal interferon. Echinacea is an herb that has been proven effective in reducing viral activity. It also stimulates the immune system, and some people with fatigue who take it have noticed improved energy and stamina. Take 15 drops of echinacea tincture three times a day.

Consider super herbs. Ginseng and ginkgo are two powerful herbs that tend to energize people. Because these are usually expensive herbs, get standardized extracts of them so that you know precisely what and how much you are getting of the herb.

Consider super foods. Spirulina and bee pollen are nutrition-rich super foods. Some people claim that they get a big boost in energy from them. Blend one teaspoon of each into a juice, or take a couple capsules of each with a meal.

Your energy should mushroom. Shiitake or reishi mushrooms can strengthen your immune system and increase your energy. Take as directed on the label.

Take advantage of your slowed-down condition. Savor every short-term activity. Appreciate the little things in life. Read a paragraph and truly digest it. Meditate for 20 minutes, and try to do it twice a day. Try yoga; the exercises won't exhaust you, and they can help to oxygenate your cells in a gentle way.

Try aggressive rest therapy. The body is better able to heal itself during sleep. Get an adequate amount of sleep, and take naps as needed during the day without feeling guilty about it. As you close your eyes, visualize your sleeping and napping times as healing experiences.

Try aggressive emotional rest, too. Don't waste your energy on negative emotions that simply drain you and add to your fatigue. When you are fatigued, you tend to complain about it; this is expected, but watch yourself to make certain you don't dwell on complaining. Also, try not to get sucked into other people's emotional dramas, unless you can get in and out without exhausting yourself. You have enough of your own dramas to worry about right now.

Forgive yourself, forgive others. When you're fatigued, you may not be able to accomplish your regular "can do" things. Allow yourself to lick your wounds and heal yourself. Forgive others who may not understand why you don't have the energy to do things as you've done them in the past.

Take your job and love it. If you truly love your work, it can be the best energizer for you. Anything that gives your life purpose and meaning is highly therapeutic. If you're unable to change jobs and work at something you really feel passionate about, find something in your job that you love.

14
Headaches (Migraine)

"The bigger a man's head, the worse his headache."
— PERSIAN PROVERB

What most people think are migraine headaches are really tension headaches. "Real" migraine headaches are usually associated with nausea or vomiting and tend to be preceded by seeing flashes of light, zigzags, blind spots, or stars. Doctors call these preceding visual symptoms "auras," which are not nearly as much fun or as practical as what New Age people refer to as auras (and the nausea is no fun at all). Migraines are often triggered by psychological stress, but distinct from tension headaches, migraines tend to begin after a stressed person is finally able to relax; then that "relaxing" weekend or vacation becomes relaxation hell. During a migraine headache, blood vessels initially become overly constricted and then abnormally widened. You usually experience this pain on one side of the head, which can make you feel lopsided. Timber!

Other triggers of migraines are sleeping too long, bright

lights, too much time between eating, and fluctuations in hormone levels (some women get migraines during menstruation or during ovulation). Certain foods, drinks, and drugs can also set off a migraine.

When a migraine is triggered, your head seems to explode. The pain can feel like there's an alien being inside the head that is trying to get out through the eyes or the forehead. It can feel as though there's someone knocking at the door, inside your head, and there is no one home to answer, so the knocking unceasingly continues. These are but some of the experiences felt inside the torture chamber of migraine sufferers' heads.

Some migraine headache sufferers experience symptoms that warn them of an impending headache. Most commonly, these warning symptoms are disturbances of vision, slurred speech, dizziness, "floating" visual images, and weakness or numbness on one side of the body. If you are having a headache or any of these warning symptoms (and if the symptoms do not stem from drinking alcohol), consider these strategies.

Loosen up. The late family therapist Virginia Satir once said, "If you have a stiff body, it's no wonder you're numb upstairs." So, loosen your body. Try to move every joint in your body, one joint at a time, through its full range of motion. If you have access to a pool, do it in water.

Around the head in a couple of minutes. While sitting up, relax the head and allow it to be as limp as possible, letting your chin touch or almost touch your upper chest. Rotate the head clockwise very slowly several times, and then counterclockwise the same number of times.

Exercise to exorcise your migraine. Exercise can be effective in preventing a migraine. When you feel a headache coming on, exercise it out of you. If it hurts to move too much, however, try gentle motion exercise such as yoga, tai chi, or slow swimming.

Headache-few with feverfew. Research published in the British medical journal *The Lancet* has shown that the herb feverfew is very helpful for vascular headaches. Scientists have proven that feverfew stops the blood platelets from releasing an excessive amount of serotonin, which tends to lead to migraine headaches. The preparations used in these studies are usually 0.2% parthenolide content or 25 mg of the freeze-dried pulverized leaves taken twice daily. These doses may prevent a migraine, while higher doses may be necessary to treat an acute attack (0.6% of parthenolide daily or one to two grams of the ground herb).

Are foods giving you a headache? Certain foods can trigger a vascular headache. No food will cause *everybody's* headache, but many migraine sufferers cannot deny that there are foods that do aggravate their problem. The most common offenders are: nuts, chocolate, coffee, sauerkraut, wheat, cheese and other dairy products, hot dogs, luncheon meats that contain nitrites, citrus, MSG, and alcohol (especially red wine). Sadly, many salad bars keep vegetables fresh looking by using sulfites, chemicals that can cause or exacerbate a headache.

As above, so below. The congestion you feel in your head may be connected, in part, to the congestion you feel in your gut. (Read the Constipation section.)

So below, as above. Stand on your head or shoulders, or hang upside down. Remember to breathe regularly. This exercise stimulates circulation and helps to break up some head congestion. Do this for a minute, and then with practice, try to extend it. To avoid possible head or neck injury, you should learn the proper position from a yoga book or yogi teacher. Don't do it if you have back problems or if it makes your head hurt too much.

Hot bathing and cold water torture. Fill a bathtub with hot water, and add several teaspoons of Epsom salts. Soak in the tub for 10 to 20 minutes, and melt and relax in this comfort. Dry off, drain the water, get back in the tub, and turn on the cold shower, allowing the cold water to spray your feet, knees, legs, back, torso, and head for three minutes. Dry off, dress in warm bedclothes, and relax in bed. This strategy is not for everyone, because some people are hypersensitive to heat and/or cold when they have headaches. Those people who can stand to do this hot and cold bathing will reap the benefits of improved circulation and reduced head congestion and pain.

Learn to circulate. With the aid of biofeedback, you can learn to directly affect blood circulation in your body, including the head congestion associated with a migraine headache. Courses in biofeedback are often available at community colleges, hospitals, and health centers.

Magnesium magic. Magnesium relaxes the constriction of blood vessels and helps to lower blood pressure. Some studies have shown that 200 mg of magnesium helps relieve migraines. Consider taking magnesium, preferably magnesium asparate or citrate, two or three times a day with meals.

Have sex! Although some people use headaches as an excuse for not having sex, a researcher at Southern Illinois University has found that sex may actually provide some relief for migraine sufferers. The researcher found that the more intense an orgasm, the more relief was obtained. There are, however, serious side effects to this strategy (seriously wonderful side effects!).

One ineffective idea. Two-thirds of all people who suffer from migraines come from a family of fellow sufferers. Because changing one's parents is not a one-minute strategy, it is best to consider the previous methods (also see the next tension on Tension Headaches).

15
Headaches
(Tension)

"When the head aches,
all the members partake of the pain."
—FROM *DON QUIXOTE*, BY CERVANTES

A pproximately 90 percent of headaches are tension headaches, but perhaps they should be called "tension neck- and backaches" because it's the tightening of the neck and back muscles that usually creates the head pain.

Tension headaches seem to be an equal-opportunity affliction. They can be caused by almost any type of stress: too much or too little exertion, too much or too little excitement, too hot or too cold temperatures, too much or too little sleep, too erect or too limp posture, too much or too little food, and so on.

Tension headaches can lead to irresponsible behavior, which can, actually, have a real practical value. You may tell your spouse, "I can't do the dishes, honey." You may tell your employer, "I can't finish that project." You may tell your children, "Shut up and stop having fun." This selfish

111

behavior might lead you to rest and take care of your headache. Sometimes it seems that a headache is nature's way of getting you to relax.

If, however, your teeth are clenched so tightly that people think you're doing a Clint Eastwood impersonation, if your neck is so tight that U.S. Steel wants to patent this musculature, and if your eyeballs hurt when you move them, then you are paying the price of not resting and enjoying yourself enough. You now have some catch-up to do.

If your eyes are not cooperating with you because of a headache, get someone to read the following strategies to you.

Don't relax . . . at least not yet. An effective technique for reducing tension headaches is to tighten muscles in the head, neck, and jaw for five to ten seconds . . . and then release them. You may find that you will be able to achieve a deeper level of relaxation from this simple exercise.

Get in touch with the temples. Remember the old aspirin commercials showing a furrow-browed man with an awful headache? As you may recall, he is seen massaging his temples. There are important acupressure points at the temples that are often effective for relieving tension. Place four fingers

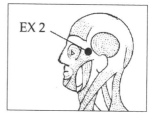

EX 2

(not the thumb) along both temples, and do a circular massaging motion. Massage for a minute . . . and call me in the morning.

Head to acupressure. The head and neck are full of invaluable acupressure points that can release tension when they are pressed firmly. Search your head and neck for "hot" points—that is, points that seem to be sensitive to pressure. Press them for at least five seconds, relax for five seconds, and repeat several times.

Your head is in your hands. There is an acupuncture point just barely below the nail of your middle finger. If your pain is primarily on one side, then press the point on that side's hand, and if on both sides, then alternate pressing each hand.

Pretend to yawn. Chew a bit. Relax that jaw! If the jaw is tense, muscles in the head and neck can impede blood flow to the head and aggravate tension headaches.

Hot flannel. Apply hot (not too hot!) flannel to the nape of the neck. It can help relax your neck and relieve tension there.

Roll your head. Roll your pillow into a "log" shape, and place it under the neck with your head hanging over the edge. Roll your head back and forth, and also let it hang over the edge of the pillow while you relax. If this is done at the beginning of a tension headache, it can sometimes prevent it from getting worse.

Run from your headache. Exercise can help loosen you up and release head, neck, and back tension. Exercising outside, as long as it is not too smoggy, carries the extra benefit of allowing you to breathe fresh air.

Take a coffee break? Drinking coffee is known to cause headaches in many people. It is also common to experience headaches while going through caffeine withdrawal. Don't drink coffee; break away from it.

Head for the herbs. Various herbal teas can help you relax. Place a tablespoon each of chamomile and skullcap into a cup of boiling water, and let it steep for five minutes. Another good combination of herbs is one teaspoon each of hops and peppermint, and two teaspoons each of chamomile, rosemary, and wood betony.

Support your head. Evening primrose oil and gingko help improve circulation to the head and can help reduce headache pain. Take 500 mg of primrose oil and gingko tablets three times a day.

*A **bright idea.*** Cool-white fluorescent lights, which are commonly used in many businesses, give some people headaches. Ask your employer to help enhance worker health and productivity by replacing these bulbs with full-spectrum lighting.

Color yourself pain-free. Close your eyes and imagine a cool color pervading your head and neck. Choose whatever color is soothing to you. This cooling color should be moving and sweeping around. Don't let it stagnate. Research has shown that color does affect brain chemistry and behavior. Color therapy is not simply something for those who are interested in fashion; it also has potentially profound healing effects.

No noise is good noise. Excessive noise can irritate anyone. Avoid loud music or being in situations where there is a lot of noise. Avoid yelling at people to ask them not to be so noisy!

Check if your head is on straight. "_____ (fill in your name here), sit up straight!" Improper posture can stress neck and back muscles. If your office desk, the seat in your car, or any chair in your house doesn't give you good support, do something about it.

Learn to listen to your body. One of the most common and effective uses of biofeedback is teaching people how to treat headaches by learning how to consciously relax the head, neck, and jaw muscles. After you learn some basics of your ability to affect your own body, you can learn to do so without being hooked up to a machine.

Watch* Candid Camera *reruns. Laughter releases tension. You may laugh your headache off.

Play a different game. Tension headaches can result from an overcompetitive personality. Create win-win situations. Appreciate the art of losing. Honor the quality of the performance, not simply the first prize.

Consider the various Migraine Headache strategies. The methods in the previous section may benefit you, too. Experiment with them.

16

Heart Disease

"The trouble with heart disease is that the first symptom is often hard to deal with: sudden death."
—MICHAEL PHELPS

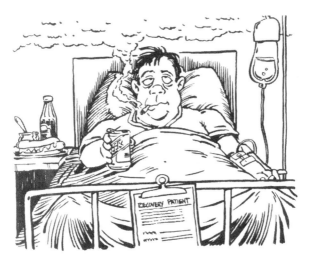

Bypass surgery tends to bypass the problem.

It is heartbreaking to realize that heart disease is the number-one killer of men and women in Western civilization, especially because we are primary accomplices to this crime. Our high-fat diet, sedentary lifestyle, stressful environment, and various vices—tobacco, alcohol, and many recreational drugs—harden the heart and its arteries and increase the risk of heart disease and early death. Although we don't get jail time for these crimes, we suffer in other ways.

In addition to these various negative influences that weigh heavily upon the heart, we also tend to suffer from a deficiency in the positive experiences that lighten the heart's load. Love, joy, pleasure, humor, and other enriching feelings not only help us feel joyfully connected with others, but also may help keep open the arteries and veins so that our circulatory system is able to interconnect with all parts of our body in a healthy way.

There are many influences that increase or decrease your risk of heart disease, but, like so many issues in medicine and science, there is probably more controversy than agreement on what exactly individuals should do to help themselves live longer, healthier lives. Even when the "experts" agree on some issue, it is always uncertain how long this agreement will last. There was, for instance, some consensus that salt was a significant factor in causing hypertension. Recent research, however, has shown that salt does not lead to hypertension in most people—but only in those who are, for unknown reasons, sensitive to it.

Despite the various controversies and ambiguities of medical science, it is instructive to remember the words of author Norman Cousins, who said, "No one knows enough to be a pessimist about their own health." On this optimistic note, I encourage you to consider the following strategies, which may not only help you lead a longer, healthier life, but also a more joyful one.

For people on conventional antihypertensive drugs who choose to use one or more of the strategies below, make certain to watch your blood pressure carefully, because it may get too low. You may need to stop trying to heal yourself . . . or better yet, you may need to reduce your conventional medication.

If you don't use it, you lose it. Exercise! Medical associations usually encourage heart patients to consult with their physician before beginning an exercise program. Considering the therapeutic value of exercise upon the heart and a person's overall health, it seems wiser to see a physician if you do *not* choose to exercise. A sedentary lifestyle should only be available by prescription to people with a serious disorder. The best exercises for a healthy heart are those that exercise the long muscles, such as jogging, swimming, rowing, walking, and various running sports. Isometrics and weightlifting, on the other hand, can raise your blood pressure and should be avoided.

Walk, walk, walk. Although this is more of an "or so" strategy than a minute strategy, new research has shown that people who walk at least three hours per week at three to four miles per hour (this is steady walking, not "mall walking") have a diminished chance of getting heart disease. The additional good news is that you can read this book and walk at the same time!

Lighten up. Jog with a 50-pound backpack. After one minute, you will discover how much extra stress this extra baggage places on you and your heart. If you're not at or near your optimal weight, you are continually stressing your heart. One option: If you simply maintain your present calorie intake for one year and increase your activity level by walking one mile a day, you will lose ten pounds.

Pretend you're Italian. Put garlic on everything! Garlic has been shown to prevent the formation of clots, lower blood pressure, reduce plaque formation, and even reverse established atherosclerosis. Garlic also boosts the high-density lipoproteins (the good guys!). If you cook with garlic, recent research has shown that it has considerably more health benefits if you cut fresh garlic and leave it sitting out for at least ten minutes before cooking with it. Brave people or hermits should try eating fresh cloves, while others can purchase the capsulated garlic (just make certain to get garlic pills from reputable companies).

Sow your oats (and other sources of fiber). The water-soluble fiber from various grains, especially oats, is able to get into your arteries, break down cholesterol, and do some Roto-rooter cleaning. Psyllium, the primary ingredient in many fiber-rich products, has been found to significantly lower serum cholesterol. Other good sources of fiber are most whole grains and legumes, especially wheat, brown rice, lentils, and dried peas. Most fresh fruits and vegetables, especially apples, figs, broccoli, and Brussels sprouts are also fiber-rich.

A carrot a day will keep heart disease away. Carrots are high in beta-carotene, which has been found to prevent coronary artery disease. Other vegetables rich in beta-carotene are spinach, cabbage, and orange and yellow fruits. In addition to eating these vegetables, it is highly recommended to take 50 mg of beta-carotene a day.

Hearty supplements. The following supplements can be helpful to the heart: 100–200 IU of vitamin E three times a day, 1,000–3,000 mg of vitamin C, 100 mcg a day of selenium, 200 mcg of chromium chloride, and 500–1,000 mg of calcium (calcium is especially important for postmenopausal women). Magnesium and potassium supplements are particularly important if you're taking diuretics.

Cooperate with Co-Enzyme Q10. Co-enzyme Q10 improves heart muscle oxygenation and is particularly important for people with hypertension, angina, congestive heart failure, and mitral valve prolapse. CoQ10, as its friends call it, is also an essential component of metabolic processes involved in energy production in the cell. This is a very helpful supplement for people with many kinds of heart disease. Take 60–100 mg per day.

Niacin to the rescue, too. Niacin has been shown to lower the amount of bad cholesterol in the body and increase the amount of good cholesterol. A decrease of 10 to 25 percent in cholesterol is common in people who either take niacin alone or with other supplements. It is recommended to increase the amount of niacin slowly. Start with 100 mg of niacin three times a day for the first three days, increase to 200 mg three times a day for the next three days, and then increase by 100 mg per dose every three days until you are taking 1,000 mg per dose three times a day. Niacin should not, however, be taken by people with liver disease, and it is best to take this supplement under the care of a physician.

Don't just supplement yourself. Just adding various supplements to a high-fat, high-cholesterol diet is not effective. The most effective way to get the most out of vitamins is to complement their use with a healthier, lower-fat diet.

Cut the fat out. To a person with heart disease, cutting down slightly on fats only marginally slows down the disease process. To make real headway and "heartway," it is necessary to significantly cut down on fats, especially animal fats. It is particularly important to avoid eating late at night because then whatever fat you eat goes into the bloodstream at a time when your circulation has slowed down, leading to increased chances of arterial blockage.

There are good fats in this world! Essential fatty acids from flaxseed, evening primrose, or borage can lower cholesterol and triglyceride levels. Take one to two tablespoons per day. There are also essential fatty acids in certain fish, especially salmon, mackerel, and herring.

Giggle with guggul. Guggul *(Commiphora mukul)* is one of India's most well-known and respected herbal remedies. A couple of studies have shown that it can lower cholesterol and triglycerides. Take 500 mg per day.

Get yeasted. Red yeast *(Monascus purpureus)*, which is cultivated on rice, contains several important chemicals that help the body form the good cholesterol (HDL) and reduce production of the bad kind (LDL). Whether you take this in bulk or in pill form, it can be helpful. In pill form, it is recommended that you take four 600 mg capsules of standardized red yeast per day (one such product is called Cholestin).

It's tea time! Black tea contains tannic acid, an astringent compound that has been found to lower cholesterol. Do not, however, brew your black tea too long, for taking larger doses of it can lead to indigestion.

To aspirin or not to aspirin. Although recent research has shown the benefits of aspirin to the heart, other research has shown that aspirin can have detrimental effects on the immune system. Aspirin not only blocks the anti-clotting effects of hormonelike chemicals called prostaglandins, but it also inhibits the infection-fighting action of the prostaglandins. There are safer means of preventing heart disease. If, however, you do decide to use aspirin to prevent blood clotting and a heart attack, take half an aspirin a day.

Don't mix grapefruit juice and calcium channel blockers. Grapefruit juice can dramatically increase the concentration of calcium channel blockers in the bloodstream and cause a medical emergency. Be careful about such "mixed" drinks.

Relax and relax again. Do whatever activities relax you, and consider using tried-and-true strategies such as meditation, yoga, and biofeedback that can help you reach deeper states of relaxation. Just as many people go to aerobics classes as a way to maintain a fitness program, it is also helpful to go regularly to yoga, meditation, or relaxation classes for the expert teaching and group support that will keep you on the program.

Relaxation is only a breath away. Proper breathing is not only relaxing, it can help oxygenate the blood and improve heart function. Most people breathe primarily with their chest, which encourages rapid, shallow breathing. A deeper and more relaxing breath is obtained through abdominal breathing. To practice abdominal breathing, sit comfortably with your back straight. Place one hand on your chest and the other on your abdomen. Breathing in through your nose, notice the hand on your abdomen rise, while the hand on your chest hardly moves. Exhale as much as possible, even contracting your abdominal muscles so that they slightly massage internal organs. Breathe in again through your nose, and repeat this process for a couple of minutes several times a day. Although this type of breathing will feel uncomfortable at first, doing it more frequently will teach you to breathe more deeply, helping you to relax more fully and improve your health.

Berry good. The hawthorn berry is one of the most common prescriptions made by German doctors to treat people with high blood pressure and angina. It has been shown to reduce blood pressure, lower cholesterol, and prevent deposits of cholesterol on arterial walls. This herb is available in pill and liquid extract forms. Take two capsules twice a day of the pill form, or take 20 to 40 drops twice a day of the liquid form. Consider also take cayenne pepper and/or ginger, preferably in pill form, to help distribute the healing effects of the hawthorn berries throughout your circulatory system.

Get hot, get cool. Stimulate circulation by alternating hot and cool showers. Do three minutes of each twice. As your heart and your courage strengthen, try using even cooler and hotter water.

Try pleasure therapy. Do whatever things you truly love—not just because it feels good, but also because it's therapeutic.

The healing power of work. Work satisfaction is invaluable to a healthy heart. If your work is fulfilling you, this satisfaction warms the heart and lowers blood pressure. Research has also shown that people whose jobs are not secure are more apt to have higher levels of serum cholesterol and higher rates of heart attack.

Acknowledge fear, and release it. Fear is a primordial survival defense; it prepares a person for fight or flight. However, fear also raises blood pressure, and if you experience it for a prolonged period of time, it can lead to hypertension. Because we sometimes feel fear when neither a fight- or-flight response is appropriate, we are bottling up powerful emotions and disturbing our health. If you try to ignore your fears, they fester, while acknowledging them is the first step that helps bring light to the shadow. As Gandolf, one of the heroes in *The Hobbit*, once said, "We must go in the direction of our greatest fear, for therein lies our only hope." Because fear often rises its head when we ignore its roots, seeking to understand it helps to release it.

17

Hemorrhoids

"Expect poison from standing water."
— WILLIAM BLAKE

Williams Blake's words were not intended to provide insight linking constipation and hemorrhoids, and yet, with apologies to the poet, it can be said (less poetically) that the stagnant waters of constipation create the breeding grounds for various health problems, including hemorrhoids.

Hemorrhoids occur when the veins at the anus are overly stretched as a result of excessive pressure, a condition that is aggravated from straining during a bowel movement. These bulging veins can occur at the anus wall or the lower bowel. It is somewhat appropriate that the old term for them was "piles." When this bulging occurs in the lower bowel, the hemorrhoid is not visible to the eye and is thus called a "blind hemorrhoid." (If I were ever reincarnated as a hemorrhoid, I'd prefer to be a deaf, dumb, and blind hemorrhoid.) A third type of hemorrhoid is one that is prolapsed; this is a blind hemorrhoid that forms clots that prevent it from receding. This type of hemorrhoid is particularly painful.

Hemorrhoids are one of the most common afflictions in Western civilization. More than half of all Americans will suffer from this undignified malady at least once in their life. When you consider the great number of people who experience hemorrhoids, it is surprising that there isn't a "Hemorrhoid Support Group" or the like.

Obesity, inactivity, frequent use of laxatives, and anal intercourse can contribute to hemorrhoids. The most common symptom is rectal bleeding, which is usually discovered by noticing blood on the toilet paper or blood-streaked stools. Such bleeding can be initially frightening, but rectal bleeding from a hemorrhoid is not a serious condition; at worst, it can be seriously embarrassing. Hemorrhoids can also be a pain in the butt, given the soreness, burning, and itching, although many people do not experience any pain there at all.

Surgery is sometimes performed on people with severe cases. Ligation surgery uses small rubber bands to tie off the hemorrhoids (what a fashion statement this can be!). Cryosurgery is a method of freezing the hemorrhoids and is considerably less painful (you just need to be certain that your doctor freezes the right things down there). Laser surgery is the latest development. The infrared light from the laser shrinks those suckers, causing them to clot and later be reabsorbed into rectal tissue (that's good because you don't want that hemorrhoidal disease circulating throughout your body—a scary thought).

However, such drastic treatments don't change the stagnant waters within the person that led to hemorrhoids in the first place. It has been said that "a hatchet is a good thing, but not with which to eat soup." Likewise, surgery is a good thing, but ... people with hemorrhoids who do not stand up to do something to heal themselves may be forced to sit on their problem. Here are some strategies to consider before the hatchet.

Read the Constipation chapter! Eat your fiber first, but don't overdue it, because this can lead to excessive bloating, gas, and even diarrhea (adding insult to injury).

Water yourself. Drink lots of fluids, especially water. If you don't, that extra fiber you should be taking may actually aggravate your constipation.

Ice up. Apply an ice cube through a cloth for 30 seconds or so. This won't cure you, but it will provide some temporarily relief.

Witch hazel isn't a witch. Witch hazel is an herb *(Hamamelis)* that is a tried-and-true folk remedy for hemorrhoids. Distilled witch hazel is available at most drugstores and is applied externally. Witch hazel can also be taken as a suppository. It is also available as a homeopathic ointment in many health food stores and some pharmacies.

Don't just sit there. It may be karmic justice that it is sometimes painful to sit when a person has hemorrhoids. Since this condition can be precipitated by physical inactivity, the discomfort from sitting is a painfully clear message that you should get off your duff and exercise.

Don't read on the throne. Because people who are constipated sometimes take a long time to defecate, they often bring a book or a magazine with them. Although reading may help pass the time, it doesn't necessarily help anything else pass, and may, in fact, increase sitting time. Since sitting for prolonged periods can aggravate hemorrhoids, leave *War and Peace* for your reading chair, not the toilet.

Don't stop breathing. When the going gets tough, people tend to stop breathing in their efforts to push out a stool. This straining can aggravate hemorrhoids. It is better to breathe deeply and evenly during bowel movements.

Schizophrenic bathing. Take a hot bath and a cold bath—alternating each for 20 minutes. Ideally, you should take a Sitz bath—a bath in which only your lower abdomen, hips, and buttocks are immersed. The alternating of hot and cold water stimulates circulation. Some people add Epsom salts to the water, although there isn't any evidence yet that this is more helpful.

Internal lubrication. Flaxseed oil can help soften your stools. Take one or two tablespoons daily.

Internal herbal relief. Stoneroot *(Collinsonia canadensis)* and Pilewort *(Lesser celandine)* are herbs that have been used for thousands of years for hemorrhoids. If it was good for you in a past life, it may be good for you today. Take two capsules of either of these herbs with a glass of water twice a day, or place one ounce of the herb in one pint of boiling water. Let it steep and drink a half cup twice a day.

External herbal relief. Yarrow *(Millefolium)* and goldenseal *(Hydrastis)* are both astringent herbs, which means that they can constrict the bulging tissue of hemorrhoids. Steep yarrow, and then add a teaspoon of goldenseal powder. Take a cotton swab and apply it directly to the hemorrhoid.

Supplementary relief. Take 1,000–2,000 mg of vitamin C, 400 IU of vitamin E, 25,000 IU of vitamin A and potassium, 600 mg of calcium, and 300 mg of magnesium. Vitamins C and E strengthen capillaries; vitamin A improves the integrity of cell walls; and potassium, calcium, and magnesium are vital for muscle health. If much blood is lost from the hemorrhoid, take 10–15 mg of iron, 400 mcg of folic acid, and 1–4 mcg of B_{12}.

Take preparation H-omeopathic. Homeopathic *Hamamelis* (witch hazel) 12 or 30 is good for bleeding hemorrhoids, which cause a bruised soreness, possibly with pulsations felt in the rectum. *Aesculus* (horse chestnut) 12 or 30 is good for hemorrhoidal pain that worsens when standing or walking, usually without bleeding and sometimes with a backache. This medicine is commonly given to women who have hemorrhoids during menopause. *Pulsatilla* (windflower) 12 or 30 is good for blind hemorrhoids with itching and sticking pains, especially in pregnant women. *Nux vomica* (poison nut) 12 or 30 is good for blind hemorrhoids in people who have frequent ineffectual urgings for a bowel movement, often from abuse of laxatives or various drugs.

A yogic tune-up! Tone your abdomen by lying on your back with your feet flat on the floor. Place your feet close to your buttocks, and lift your hips off the floor. Take a complete in- and outbreath while remaining in the raised position. Raise and lower yourself six times in this way.

Lift properly. Because improper lifting strains rectal tissue and leads to or aggravates hemorrhoids, learn the proper way to lift: Bend your knees, avoid bending your back, and don't lift beyond your strength or for great distances.

Some things to not do. Avoid prolonged use of laxatives or mineral oil (even herbal laxatives). Avoid using ointments and suppositories for more than 14 days unless your condition is medically monitored. Avoid scratching the irritated area, and avoid heavy lifting.

18

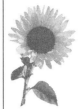

Herpes

"Sleep, riches, and health,
to be truly enjoyed, must be interrupted."
—FROM *FLOWER, FRUIT, AND THORN,*
BY JEAN PAUL RICHTER (1796)

Herpes was once considered the modern "scarlet letter," until the AIDS epidemic spread and stole its thunder. Although this sexually transmitted disease is no longer a "media star," herpes is as common as it was several years ago.

Herpes is caused by a virus, and once a person is infected, the virus gets into nerve cells where the immune system cannot find or get rid of it. Although you may be horrified by this prospect, it is generally not as traumatic as it sounds. Many people who get infected experience only a single eruption and rarely or never get another, and it is common for people to have decreasing outbreaks over time. It is also good news to hear that outbreaks rarely occur in people over 50 years old (can you wait that long?). Even for those individuals who get more frequent eruptions, modern medical drugs and some emerging natural therapies can be very effective in reducing the frequency and intensity of outbreaks.

Herpetic eruptions most commonly occur on the lips of the mouth or on the genitals, although different viruses cause them. Herpes in the mouth is caused by herpes virus Type 1, and herpes in the genitals by herpes virus Type 2, but strangely enough, mouth herpes is referred to both as a "cold sore" and a "fever blister." Perhaps people can't figure out if this eruption is too cold or too hot.

Although the herpes condition can be relatively benign, it can cause complications when a pregnant woman with an herpetic outbreak gives birth, because the infant can get a potentially fatal infection. Herpes has also been linked to later onset of cervical cancer, so women with herpes should get Pap smears regularly. Furthermore, if herpes is spread to the eyes, it can lead to blindness. People who get such infections may be rubbing their eyes the wrong way, or they may be looking for love in all the wrong places.

Perhaps the most frequent complication arising from herpes is the guilt and general anxiety that too often accompany it. Those infected with herpes often observe that they are more prone to outbreaks during times of psychological stress, so the more they reduce this extra baggage of anxiety, the less they have to experience the herpes.

New medical research has developed a herpes vaccine,

but for mice only (perhaps this explains why Mickey and Minnie smile so much). Although this vaccine may not be valuable for current sufferers, such advances may be invaluable in the future. In the meantime, here are some strategies to help alleviate some of the pain and discomfort of herpes.

Freeze 'em out. If you apply ice to herpes sores as soon as they erupt, you can sometimes prevent them from getting worse.

Witch hazel to the rescue. Apply distilled witch hazel to sores to help dry them out. Another herb that can dry out herpes blisters is tincture of myrrh.

A blow dryer job. Another way to dry out moist blisters is to use a blow dryer, but be careful not to irritate the sores by drying them too long or too closely.

Take tea and see. Pour hot water over a black tea bag—just enough to moisten it. Let it sit without contact with the hot water for a couple minutes to cool down, and then place the tea bag on the sore. Black tea has tannic acid that not only can reduce the pain, but is also astringent and can help constrict the skin.

Take a tea tree break. Tea tree oil is a powerful natural antiseptic which, when applied directly onto the sore, can dry it out and heal it. Use a Q-Tip to dab it, and avoid placing too much of the oil on the sore. If there is too much stinging, consider diluting the oil with water. Avoid placing tea tree oil near the eyes.

Red wine will make it fine. Researchers have found that freeze-dried red wine has concentrated tannins in it, which can relief the pain of herpes sores. Apply it topically with a Q-Tip. Freeze-dried red wine is available in some wine specialty shops.

Salt your wounds. Bathe in a tub in which a half cup of salt has been added. This may sting a bit at first but will soon feel comforting.

Check your aminos. Some research has shown that increasing certain amino acids and decreasing others leads to reduced and less intense herpetic eruptions. It may be worthwhile for you to determine for yourself if the following program works for you. Taken on an empty stomach, the amino acid lysine may help to inhibit herpes replication. In contrast, another amino acid, arginine, encourages herpes replication. Increase lysine by taking a supplement separate from a meal (1,000 mg a day when sores aren't active, and 2,000 mg when they are active).

It is generally recommended to avoid taking lysine longer than six months at a time.

Taken with lysine, you should also take 50 mg of vitamin B_6 and 100 mg of vitamin C, which help the body better absorb lysine. You should also consider eating more of the following foods that are lysine-rich: fish (especially shark), chicken, milk, yogurt, fresh vegetables, eggs, Brewers yeast, soybeans, and legumes. Because sugar, fats, and protein can inhibit absorption of lysine, it is wise to reduce their consumption. Foods rich in arginine that should be avoided are nuts, chocolate, seeds, cottonseed oil, coconut, macaroni, oats, wheat germ, whole wheat bread, and coffee.

External vitamins. Prick a cap of vitamin E, and apply the liquid directly to the sore every four hours.

Internal vitamins and minerals. Beta-carotenes inhibit viruses and augment the immune system; take 100,000 IU per day (if pregnant, don't take more than 10,000 IU per day). Vitamin E helps decrease pain and shortens the time of herpetic eruption; take 400 IU per day. Zinc has been shown to inhibit herpes virus replication in vitro (in test tubes). Take 15 mg of zinc picolinate per day, and apply zinc sulphate solution externally 0.25% solution three times a day.

The fungus among us. Maitake, shiitake, and reishi mushrooms all have antiviral and immuno-enhancing properties. They are readily available at most health food stores. Take them as directly on the label.

Don't touch yourself. Avoid touching your sores, and if you do, wash your hands carefully afterwards so that you don't spread the virus to other parts of your body, especially your eyes.

Let your skin breathe. Wear natural-fiber clothing that allows skin to breathe, and avoid pants (especially underwear) that are too tight. Also, avoid applying petroleum jelly and antibiotic ointments that inhibit the ability of your skin to breathe and can slow the healing of herpes blisters.

Soothing herbs. Tinctures of *Calendula* (marigold) and *Hypericum* (St. John's wort) are both soothing herbs that can reduce some of the inflammation of a herpes sore. These tinctures should be slightly diluted (one part tincture to two parts water).

The healing powers of poison ivy. Believe it or not, poison ivy in a homeopathic dose is often effective in treating people with herpes. Because poison ivy can cause blisters that resemble herpes, utilizing the principles of homeopathy, very small doses of poison ivy can help heal them. Use *Rhus tox* (poison ivy) 6 or 30 three times a day for two or three days. Another helpful homeopathic medicine to try is *Natrum mur* (salt) 6 or 30.

Avoid heavy sex. Even when you do not have an eruption, vigorous or long-lasting sex can irritate the genitals and cause eruptions. This is particularly a problem if partners are not adequately lubricated.

Condomize. The use of condoms is an important way to prevent infecting others. Because it is possible to spread herpes even when you don't have an obvious sore, it is best to use them every time you have sex (there are, of course, a few other good reasons for using condoms, too).

Get support. Join a herpes support group if you feel you need help in working out whatever feelings of guilt, fear, or anxiety you are experiencing as the result of your condition. If there isn't one locally, check out the Internet.

You are not herpes. You may *have* herpes, but you are *not* herpes. Avoid identifying yourself, even subconsciously, as a herpes sufferer. This attitude may not cure your herpes, but it will reduce the anxiety that tends to accompany the outbreaks.

19

indigestion

*"Indigestion is charged by God
with enforcing morality in the stomach."*
—VICTOR HUGO

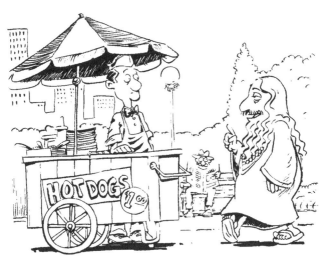

"Make me ONE with everything."
Yogi about to become ONE with indigestion.

Some people say that you are what you eat, but this bit of twisted logic is probably only seriously considered by people who eat pretzels.

Sadly enough, we do not digest all the food we eat. One might then say: You are what you assimilate. However, even this perspective is narrowly focused on food. If you are what your body takes in, are you then also what you breathe, what your skin absorbs, and what your mind thinks? If we are all this and more, mixed together, it is certainly understandable why so many people have indigestion.

Los Angeles comedian Darryl Henriques perhaps said it best when he said, "You are what you don't poop."

Indigestion is a very broad term that refers to virtually any problem related to digesting food. Most commonly, it refers to heartburn, gas, and distention of the abdomen (see the sections on Constipation, Diarrhea, Irritable Bowel Syndrome, Nausea, and Ulcers for information on each of these related conditions).

Heartburn is a misnomer, since it is not really the heart that is burning. Perhaps it's called this because it is often the food we truly love that tends to upset us, thus breaking our heart ... and our stomach. Heartburn is actually a condition in which the esophagus or stomach is irritated by too much acid from the foods eaten or from the digestive acids that are secreted to digest them. The body may slightly regurgitate the food and the acids, thereby creating some burning in the middle of the chest. Because the pain is at or near the heart, heartburn scares many people, leading them to take various over-the-counter medications that provide temporary relief. These drugs, however, offer only short-term relief and often aggravate the condition.

Stomach gas is experienced by virtually everyone, although some people are larger producers of it than others. This gas can come from the excessive swallowing of air or from the action of bacteria on the incomplete digestion of carbohydrates. Depending on where the gas is temporarily trapped, the body will release it through one orifice or another. Some people even seem to be full-blown gas refineries.

More than 2,000 years ago, Hippocrates said, "Passing gas is necessary to well-being." These may be refreshingly reassuring words to those people who regularly pass gas, but it may be less refreshing to others nearby.

In the 1960s, a classic commercial showed a man talking to his stomach, which expressed concern about the way the man was treating it and asked the man to be more sensitive to its problems. Whether you talk to your stomach or not, your stomach talks to *you*. It does so by the way it expresses its symptoms. Sometimes its message is clear and direct: "Stop eating that food." "Don't eat anymore." "Eat more slowly." At other times, it is difficult to interpret what it is saying, and you may ask yourself: *Which food should I stop eating? Why do I have gas now? That antacid worked before; why isn't it working now?*

We were all taught to speak one language, and sometimes several, but few of us have learned to understand the language of the body. And even if we know what the body is saying, we don't always pay attention. Whether we understand what our bodies are saying or not, it is worthwhile to listen. It is also important to ask the body what it means. Since the body doesn't speak English, "asking it" may mean testing it by trying to do or eat something differently and then paying attention to the reaction.

Here are several strategies to consider in your efforts to respond to your poor, abused digestive system.

Eat small. Don't get into the routine of eating three large meals a day. Your body might digest your food better when eating smaller, more frequent meals.

Slow down and chew. This is just one more instance in which your mother was right! A significant percentage of digestion, especially of carbohydrates, takes place in your mouth from juices in the saliva. If you gulp down your food, you're not giving your body enough opportunity to digest it. You should try to chew your foods until they're almost liquid in your mouth. You should even chew your drinks, especially juices and sodas. Just remember: Drink your food and chew your drinks.

Slow the fiber. Although fiber is important for digestion and elimination, too much fiber or a too-rapid increase in fiber to the diet can cause serious gas problems. The foods with the most fiber are bran, prunes, figs, whole grains, legumes, broccoli, cauliflower, onions, cabbage, and raisins.

Avoid heartburn hotel. Coffee, acidic fruits (tomatoes and grapefruits), chocolate, alcohol, nitrates, and fatty foods can irritate the lining of the esophagus and lead to heartburn. Even smoking can cause heartburn because it increases pressure at the lower end of the esophagus.

Get the right combination. Some people notice that they develop indigestion if they eat certain foods in combination. This may be true for you. Some of the most common problems are a meat dish with a starchy food, or a grain dish with dairy products. Some people also experience digestive problems when they eat one type of fruit with any other fruit or food. The good news here is that you may discover that a food that had previously caused you digestive problems may be fine as long as it is not combined with other foods.

Avoid the bubbly. Carbonated drinks and beer can create or add to a gas problem. Since you can't bottle the gas you create, it's better to avoid those drinks that can turn you into a gas refinery.

Artificial sweeteners create not-so-artificial problems. Artificial sweeteners are indigestible carbohydrates that turn your body into a gas production factory. Avoid them.

Milk can add fuel to the flames. Milk and milk products can aggravate heartburn because the body produces increased acid to digest them.

Suck up to a straw. Drinking through a straw cuts down on the air that you may be inhaling as you drink.

Bring out the charcoal. Activated charcoal tablets are invaluable for excessive flatulence, since charcoal absorbs gases.

Don't take it lying down. People with chronic heartburn should not eat while reclining or lying down. In fact, you should even avoid lying down until two or three hours after eating.

Sow your oats and drink up. Soak one tablespoon each of oatmeal and bran in a pint of water for 30 minutes. Strain and drink the water. This liquid is both nourishing and soothing to the digestive tract.

An old-time remedy. A tablespoon of apple cider vinegar

before meals is an old-time remedy for acid indigestion. A tablespoon each of apple cider vinegar and honey is great for relieving gas.

In mint condition. Peppermint and spearmint teas are soothing for many types of indigestion. Other herbal teas that are digestion helpers are chamomile, rosemary, and blackberry.

To the bitter end. Herbal bitters, often just called bitters, activate the secretion of digestive juices. Some of the most common bitters are gentian, goldenseal, and dandelion root.

More herbal help. Fennel seeds are commonly available at the counters of Indian restaurants because they are known to help people digest food better. One special recipe to augment the action of fennel is to grind it and add it to grated ginger and honey. Eat it with a spoon. It tastes great, and it's good for you. Ginger is, in particular, useful for nausea and/or vomiting. Take 2–4 g two or three times a day, or 250 mg every two or three hours. Also, slippery elm bark—1/4 of an ounce to a pint of water—is a wonderfully soothing and nourishing drink for the digestive system (but I must warn you that this mixture is rather slimy and tastes a bit weird!).

Go Italian. Garlic is invaluable for painful digestion or for flatulence.

Get infected with good bacteria. The good bacteria within yogurt and miso help the digestive process, though people who are sensitive to dairy products should avoid yogurt. The good bacteria are also readily available through various acidophilus products that come in pill or liquid form.

Get some spark. Fresh papaya and pineapple contain beneficial digestive enzymes that aid the digestive process. Consider also taking digestive enzymes in pill form, too.

The drugs made you do it. Certain prescription drugs cause indigestion. Check with your doctor about the drugs that you are taking; you may want to just say no to these drugs or switch to others.

Relieve pressure by placing pressure. While holding the different sides of the kneecap with your index finger and thumb, place your middle finger outside of the shinbone and press it for five to ten seconds. This acupuncture point is "Stomach 36," and applying pressure to it can relax the stomach and reduce indigestion. Other points listed in the accompanying graphic can also be helpful.

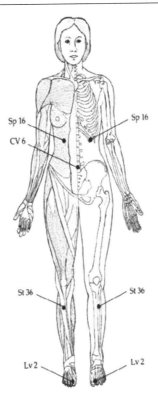

Sit-ups for health. Sit-ups improve abdominal muscle tone and can reduce excessive distention. Do them regularly.

Relax during those intimate moments. Straining during defecation can increase abdominal pressure, causing heartburn and indigestion. Take it slow and easy.

Bottle up the belching. Forced belching tends to add even more air to the stomach than it releases. Not only is forced belching ill-mannered, it isn't good for you. Ms. Manners scores again!

Release the butterflies in your stomach. Accept the anxiety, the nervousness, and the fear that you're holding in, then release it. If you need to scream, scream. If you need to jump around, jump around. If you need to talk incessantly, do so . . . but not to me.

20

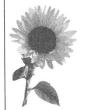

Influenza (Flu)

*"We forget ourselves and our destinies
in health, and the chief use of temporary
sickness is to remind us of these concerns."*
—RALPH WALDO EMERSON

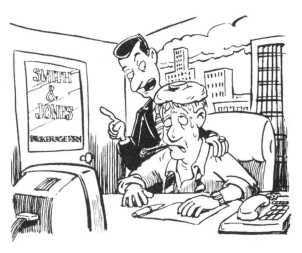

When it gets to 103 degrees, sell.

Also called "the grippe," influenza can indeed get a hold of you. It can last for three to ten days and make you feel as if a demon has taken possession of your body. You may have a fever that simulates a fire from hell, weakness as though a vampire has sucked your energy, body aches like a tin man who hasn't been oiled, nausea that makes you feel as if an alien has taken refuge in your abdomen, and a congestive headache that feels like your brain is trying to escape through your eyeballs or forehead.

Despite these horrors, the flu of yesteryear was actually a lot more serious than those of today. In fact, millions of people died during the worldwide flu epidemic of 1917–18. Today, the flu's symptoms may be as mild as a low-grade fever with minor aches and perhaps a slight headache.

Some people over 65 years of age can in fact die from influenza or from one of its complications, such as pneumonia. However, for people under 65, it is rarely a serious problem, although it can make you more susceptible to other ailments, including sinus problems, ear infections, and various respiratory complaints.

Schools and worksites are literally "flu factories" because of the flu's highly contagious nature. The increased risk of getting the flu is but another price we pay for sharing the company of others. Normally it's worth the price, but you may not think so during those horrid days in bed when the flu's hellfire consumes you.

Whatever kind of symptoms you have, the flu is no fun, and it's always worthwhile to know of specific strategies that may bring you back to life sooner. There are more than 200 viruses that cause the flu and the common cold, and because they change so frequently, vaccinations at best provide short-term prevention. In any case, there are many simple ways that you can get over the flu quickly.

An old standby. Rest, warmth, and fluids are basic to the treatment of the flu. Rest is very helpful, but if you have the energy for simple chores, you should do them just as long as you don't exhaust yourself. Lots of fluids are very important to avoid getting dehydrated and to help the body eliminate the waste products from infection. If you drink juices, it is best to dilute them in half with water.

Chicken soup. Score another one for your mother. Eating hot chicken soup has been found to have antiviral effects. A million-jillion mothers couldn't be wrong.

Try Vitamin C. Although taking vitamin C is still controversial as far as its efficacy in treating the flu, research suggests that it does have some preventive action. Since it is unlikely that any adverse side effects result from short-term high doses of vitamin C, it couldn't hurt to try this strategy. Consider taking one gram every four hours while flu symptoms are present.

Zinc the flu. Zinc lozenges are sometimes therapeutic for people with the flu due to its antiviral action. Zinc seems to be more effective in smaller than larger doses. Try not to use more than 23 mg lozenges, and avoid taking more than 150 mg per day. Don't eat citrus fruits shortly before or after zinc or they can disturb assimilation of the zinc.

Be anti-antibiotics. A virus causes the flu, and antibiotics are only helpful for bacterial infections. Because doctors sometimes feel compelled to do something for you, and since patients sometimes demand that something be done, antibiotics are occasionally prescribed for the flu, even though they don't help. Just say no!

Get down on aspirin. Aspirin is generally effective in lowering fever and reducing body aches, but it should never be used for a person with influenza. Fever is an important defense of the body in its effort to fight infection; by taking aspirin and lowering the fever, you are delaying your healing. Do you really want to do that? If you have a high fever (103°F or higher) with much aching, and if other strategies are not working rapidly enough, consider taking acetaminophen (Tylenol) for temporary relief. Although it is a drug, it is safer than aspirin.

Give yourself a sponge bath. A sponge bath can be wonderful, just like the kind your mother may have given you when you could fit in the kitchen sink. Use warm, not hot, water.

An Epson salt bath. Put three tablespoons of Epsom salts in a warm bath, and soak in it for 20 minutes.

A spicy treatment. In combination, garlic and cayenne are beneficial for treating infections. Garlic has infection-fighting properties; and cayenne is good for the blood, stimulates the heart, and helps spread the action of the garlic throughout the body. Both of these herbs are available in capsule form.

An herbal booster. Echinacea is an herb that has been shown to stimulate the immune system and have antiviral actions. At the first sign of the flu, take a dropperful of Echinacea extract, or whatever it says on the label, several times a day. Also, consider mixtures of echinacea and goldenseal, except if you are pregnant. In any case, avoid taking goldenseal for longer than seven days. You can either place the liquid herbal extracts directly in your mouth, or to increase their palatability, you can place them in ginger or chamomile tea. Echinacea and goldenseal are available singly, in combination, and in pill form, also.

Try duck soup? *Oscillococcinum* is a homeopathic medicine that is a microdose taken from the liver and heart of a duck. Although this may sound a bit like witchcraft, solid research has shown it to be an effective remedy for the flu. Biologists have discovered that 80 percent of ducks have every known influenza virus in their digestive tracts. Perhaps the homeopathic dose of the liver and heart contains helpful antibodies to the flu. Considering the fact that chicken soup has antiviral properties, it is conceivable that this condensed version of duck soup is therapeutic as well.

A little dab will do ya. Two other homeopathic medicines are often effective for treating the flu, although each is primarily good for a specific pattern of symptoms. *Gelsemium* (yellow jessamine) 6 or 30 is good when your flu makes you feel tired, weak, and heavy. Your eyelids look heavy and droop. You may have the chills and a headache in the back part of the head. You have no thirst and feel great relief after you urinate.

Bryonia (wild hops) is needed if you have body aches, feel irritable, and all their pains are aggravated by any motion. You may have a headache in the front part of the head and must lie still because any motion intensifies the pain. Light touch, stooping, eating, and talking aggravate the headache, while firm pressure and lying still relieve it. You feel better in a cool room and are uncomfortable in a warm room. You have an intense thirst for cool drinks and tend to have a dry, hacking cough. Generally, it is recommended that you take the 6th or 30th potency of these medicines, usually four times a day for one to three days, stopping if symptoms abate sooner.

Aromatherapy to the rescue. To prevent the flu, gargle daily with one drop each of the essential oil from the tea tree and from the juice of a lemon. When tending to the flu, gargle with two drops each of the essential oil from the tea tree and from the geranium. If your nose and/or chest is congested, place a few drops of the essential oil from eucalyptus in a pot of recently boiled water, and breathe in the steam.

Run away from the flu. Research has shown that exercise temporarily increases the body's white blood cells, thus helping the body fend off flu viruses. This treatment, however, is better as a preventive measure than as a treatment, since people are usually too exhausted to exercise once the flu bug has struck.

21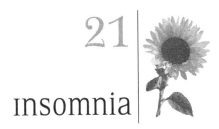

insomnia

"I hate when my foot falls asleep during the day,
because I know it's going to be up all night."
—STEVEN WRIGHT

Falling asleep can be so easy, and yet at times it can be so difficult. When insomniacs meet with narcoleptics (people who have an uncontrollable tendency to fall asleep throughout the day), each is inevitably jealous of the other's condition.

The Zenlike solution for people having difficulty falling asleep is to avoid trying so hard. However, telling an insomniac to not try to fall asleep is like telling someone who is starving to try to fast when sitting at a dinner table.

It may be reassuring to know that 15 to 25 percent of all adults suffer regularly from insomnia, but this awareness usually doesn't make falling asleep any easier. In fact, there are probably readers who will now stay up nights organizing 3:00 A.M. meetings of Insomniacs Anonymous.

While some insomniacs have difficulty falling asleep, others wake up frequently and have problems staying asleep.

Whichever problem you are experiencing, this is one whose solution cannot be easily found by sleeping on it.

The good news is that everyone does not necessarily need to have eight hours of sleep a night. Some people define themselves as "insomniacs" because they regularly sleep only five or six hours, when they should think of themselves more accurately as high-energy people who don't need a lot of sleep. Some people's body rhythms are such that their highest and most creative energy occurs late at night. The wakeful state that these people experience is not a sign of illness; it may simply be a signal—sometimes an exasperatingly loud one—that the person should use this alert time to do some creative work.

Perhaps the best way to determine if you're getting enough sleep each night is if you feel rested and refreshed upon waking. If you don't feel rested and need some help, read the next set of strategies, and you may soon be getting sleepy, very sleepy . . . very, very sleepy.

Relaxation trick #1. Hypnotize yourself. Feel total relaxation in your feet, then slowly feel the relaxation move up your body. Tell yourself that each part is feeling warm, comfortable, and relaxed. Use diaphragmatic breathing that will help relax you further (see a more detailed description of this type of breathing in the Asthma chapter).

Relaxation trick #2. Massage the soles of your feet, or preferably, have them massaged for you. This type of massage can be very relaxing.

Don't sleep tight: Relaxation trick #3. Take a warm bath in which you add a couple of drops of one or more essential oils such as orange blossom, meadowsweet, and hops.

Get in some hot water. A warm bath (or hot tub) just prior to bedtime is a great way to relax. The body actually drops in temperature after getting out of a warm bath, and a drop in temperature has been linked to feelings of sleepiness.

The melatonin solution. Many people swear by this one. Start by taking 1.5 mg of melatonin per day about two hours or less before bedtime. If this doesn't work, gradually increase the dose until you find a dose that seems to work (don't take more than 5 mg per day).

Hops to it. Hops is the herb that is used to make beer, and it is also used by herbalists to help people fall asleep. Some people brew a tea of it; others purchase the hops leaves and insert them into a pillow. "Dream pillows" are also available for purchase; these are small pillows filled with various sweet-smelling herbs that help you think sweet thoughts and dream sweet dreams.

Herbal sedatives. Steep one teaspoon each of valerian root, skullcap, and catnip for 20 minutes. One cup of this tea will relax the body and calm the mind. Another good combination of herbs is chamomile, passionflower, and hops. These herbs are available in capsule or liquid extract form, too, although drinking a warm tea of them has an additional relaxing effect.

Don't count sheep, count on sheep's wool. Wool blankets are better able to regulate skin and body temperature than synthetic blankets. A comfortable comforter may help you sleep better.

Caffeine and other stimulants lurk in unsuspecting places. Avoid caffeinated products, including colas, aspirin, diet pills, black tea, and of course, coffee. Nicotine in cigarettes is also a stimulant that will keep you up at night.

Don't go up in smoke. Nicotine, like caffeine, is a stimulant. Although the deep breathing in which people engage when they smoke can bring about feelings of relaxation, the chemical effects of nicotine act like a stimulant.

Warm milk rarely works. Despite folklore that has long

suggested that warm milk helps people sleep, research has shown that it is rarely helpful. In fact, nonfat and low-fat milk can actually stimulate the brain's activity. That said, warm or cold milk is a comfort food to some people, and it can help certain people fall asleep. See what works for you.

Avoid catnaps. Day naps should be avoided if you have problems with insomnia. Save your best 40 winks for nighttime.

Exercise earlier in the day, and avoid it at night. A well-exercised body is less likely to experience insomnia, except when exercise is done within two hours of bed-time. Late-night aerobic activity can generate too much energy to allow you to fall asleep easily.

Bedrooms are for sleeping. Avoid using your bedroom for stressful activities such as paying bills or doing work. Let your bedroom be a soothing, quiet, and relaxing place to be at all times.

Create a sleep ritual. When it's time for sleep, close the shades, get into your special bedclothes, brush your teeth, turn off the lights, and fluff the pillow. Mentally scan your body, and sense where you feel tension. Tighten it and then relax it. Take a couple of slow, deep breaths. You may also want to make certain that you are getting adequate but not too much ventilation. Do whatever other activities make you feel comfortable, secure, and relaxed.

Unmedicate yourself. Many prescription and over-the-counter drugs, including decongestants and aspirin, can disturb sleep. Talk with your doctor to see if you can reduce the dosage or change the prescription.

Rest assured, sedatives disrupt sleep. Besides being addictive, sedatives disturb deep sleep, causing you to wake up unrefreshed. Occasional use of sedatives may be worthwhile, but avoid regular use.

Don't drink your sleep away. Alcohol may make a person drowsy, but it disrupts sleep patterns and creates a fitful sleep.

Try sex. While making love can be very energizing at times, it can also be extremely relaxing, thus helping to get the sandman's attention. Don't engage in this activity if it will cause anxiety. Don't feel compelled to limit this to a one-minute healing strategy.

Try NOT to sleep. Research has suggested that insomniacs actually need less sleep than others do. Don't feel pressured to get a full eight hours every night. You may experience less anxiety about yourself and may be able to sleep better, even if you do sleep less.

Coffee as a sedative? Homeopathic doses of coffee *(Coffea)* actually help relax the mind and body. Take *Coffea* 6 or 30 thirty minutes before bedtime and then again as you get into bed. It is particularly effective for insomniacs who are physically and mentally restless.

Sweet dreams with passionflower. *Passiflora* 3 (passionflower) is perhaps the closest to a generic homeopathic medicine for insomnia in children, or the older people and for others who experience a hyperactive mind, with ideas and anxieties crowding them.

Take two mantras and call me in the morning. A mantra is usually a one- or two-syllable word that a person repeats over and over and over again. People use it as a way to calm the mind, although it can also clear the mind and encourage sleep. You don't have to use Sanskrit words as a mantra; you can use *one, God, love,* or even *sleep.*

Talk out loud. By vocally releasing the things that are bothering you, you are letting go of them. Acknowledge your anxieties, insecurities, and fears out loud. Get these emotions out and they may then let you sleep. Keeping a journal can also be very cathartic.

22
irritable Bowel syndrome

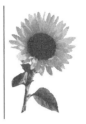

"What some call health, if purchased by perpetual anxiety about diet, isn't much better than tedious disease."
—GEORGE DENNISON PRENTICE

Irritable bowel syndrome (IBS), also known as spastic colon, can be painful, anxiety-provoking, just plain uncomfortable, and even disabling. A Jewish grandmother might describe this ailment as colon *kvetching* (a Yiddish word for "complaining"), although it's still a mystery whether one's colon is kvetching to the person or the person is kvetching to the colon (or both).

Believe it or not, IBS is the cause of more industrial absenteeism than any other condition, even more than the common cold. An estimated one in five Americans suffers from symptoms of IBS, although less than half seek professional help for it. About twice as many women suffer from IBS as men do.

Typically, people with IBS experience abdominal pain, bloating, and nausea. They also usually get diarrhea and/or constipation that may alternate. Depending on the day, an IBS sufferer doesn't know if he is coming or ... not going. And because of the pain and discomfort that some people with IBS experience, they may actually dread eating (to those of us who love to eat, this symptom makes IBS a particularly serious disease).

People with IBS typically experience poor absorption of nutrients; therefore, they need higher amounts of protein, minerals, and trace minerals. This is especially problematic for those with this condition who experience discomfort when eating.

Despite all of the troubles it brings, IBS doesn't actually involve tissue damage or inflammation in any part of the intestines. Because of this lack of physical manifestation, IBS was considered for many years to be a psychosomatic disorder. This is no longer the case. Although your emotional and mental state may affect this condition, physiological factors also can trigger this syndrome. Some people with IBS experience an exacerbation of symptoms after eating certain foods. Also, research has shown that people with IBS tend to be more sensitive to abdominal gas, leading them to feel greater stomach pains than others.

Here are some strategies to help you and your colon become less irritable and more friendly.

Find the culprit. Many IBS sufferers are allergic to one or more foods. The most common offenders are: wheat, eggs, corn, milk products, peanuts, soy, fish, fruits (especially citrus), raw vegetables, coffee, and tea. Remember: Milk is *not* for everyone! Fried and greasy foods cause problems in some people. Avoid any food or drink for at least a week, and see if you notice an improvement in your health. It is best to eliminate one food or drink at a time.

Be a detective. Keep a diary about your life and bowel habits. Pay careful attention to which events, stresses, or hormonal changes in your life may be related to bowel habits. See if you can discover those factors that trigger an attack so that you can possibly prevent future problems.

Graze. Instead of eating three relatively large-sized meals, eat five or six smaller meals throughout the day.

Your heating pad or mine? Apply a heating pad or hot water bottle to the abdomen during attacks of abdominal pain; its soothing and relaxing effects will diminish the pain.

Fiberize yourself. Eat foods rich in fiber, such as whole grains (especially wheat or oat bran), legumes, and fresh fruits and vegetables. If you're having difficulty digesting such foods, try psyllium husks, oat bran, ground flaxseeds, or one of the fiber-based products in health food stores and pharmacies.

One-a-day or more. Taking a multivitamin and mineral complex is useful in helping to supply nutrients that are not adequately absorbed from your food.

Green foods. Spirulina and chlorella are types of algae that are rich in chlorophyll, which is so beneficial for cleansing and healing the bloodstream. Alfalfa is also chlorophyll-rich and high in vitamin K, which is useful in building intestinal flora for proper digestion.

Support friendly bacteria. Eat yogurt or miso soup, or take an acidophilus supplement to help replenish the friendly bacteria that is instrument in digesting food.

Don't be artificially sweet. Sorbitol, an artificial sweetener, is known to worsen IBS because it is not easily digested. Some physicians believe that sorbitol isn't the only sweetener that can aggravate IBS. Fructose, mannitol, and other sweeteners may also be a problem because some people cannot absorb these sugars, causing them to ferment in the abdomen. Also, olestra, a fat substitute, can aggravate some people with IBS.

Cut the fat. Fats increase the muscular contractions of the colon and irritate an already irritable colon.

Drink up. Drinking lots of water or other liquids helps to replace the vital fluids lost as the result of diarrhea and helps lubricate compacted stools when you are constipated. Coffee and tea, however, should be avoided because they can irritate the colon.

Herbal soothers. Mix ½ ounce of marshmallow root, ¼ ounce of valerian root or lady's slipper, and ⅛ ounce of slippery elm. Boil this mixture in two pints of water for 15 minutes. Strain while warm. Drink ½ cup every two hours during the day.

For a mint condition. The herb peppermint is wonderfully helpful in aiding digestion. People with IBS should take enteric-coated peppermint capsules so that the peppermint oil isn't released before it reaches the colon. Take one or two capsules 20 minutes before a meal.

Don't abuse drugs. Overusing antibiotics, corticosteroids, laxatives, antacids, and antidiarrhea medications can disturb digestion and exacerbate symptoms of IBS. Consider the various natural, safer alternatives first.

Chill out. Many IBS sufferers appear cool and collected externally, while they hold much anxiety and anticipation inside. This extra holding-in effort can place extra tension on the colon. Don't be cool. Express yourself.

A little dab will do ya. Homeopathic medicines generally work most effectively when they are highly individualized to a person's unique pattern of symptoms and then prescribed in extremely small doses. However, one study on subjects with IBS showed significant improvement in symptoms when each subject was given the same remedy in an only slightly diluted dose: *Asafoetida* 3X. Take it a couple times a day, but stop taking it after a week unless you notice obvious improvement. Consider going to a professional homeopath for a more individualized and deeper-acting remedy.

Less is more. There are IBS sufferers who seem to run around as much as their stools do. It may be better, or at least less stressful, to do fewer activities in a more relaxed manner.

Say good-bye to your anxieties. One way to do so is to remember a major stress in your life that you once thought would never go away. Remember how it did? So will your present anxieties. New ones will inevitably come up, but if you have an underlying attitude that all things must pass, you can be less anxious about them and more capable of moving on.

Natural tranquilizers. Yoga and meditation are natural tranquilizers that help calm you physically, emotionally, and mentally. Try to do 20 to 30 minutes of yoga once a day, and 20 minutes of meditation twice a day.

Jog it loose. Jogging and other forms of exercise help relieve stress and release endorphins, the body's natural painkillers. Also, by improving muscle tone, you may also help improve bowel tone.

23

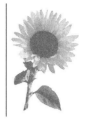

menopause

"The most creative force in the world is a menopausal woman with zest."
—Margaret Mead

As one woman friend once said, "Menopause is like a long premenstrual syndrome, and because it's the last one, it's a doozie."

Most commonly, menopause begins when a woman is between 45 and 55 years of age. Women who undergo a hysterectomy usually experience menopause shortly after surgery, and the symptoms are usually more intense. Approximately 75 percent of women experience some discomfort just prior to and during menopause, including hot flashes, vaginal dryness and itching, bladder problems, skin dryness and increased wrinkling, osteoporosis, depression, irritability, decreased libido, dizziness, insomnia, and night sweats. These symptoms can recur for up to five years.

Conventional physicians usually treat the most severe symptoms of menopause with hormone replacement therapy. Because women are encouraged to take these drugs for the rest of their life and because they can have serious side effects, women and their doctors should use them carefully and, when possible, seek safer alternatives. Whatever decision you make can and will have significant effects upon your health. Don't leave this decision just to your doctor. Talk to friends, elders, counselors, and whomever you respect. Then, make your own decision by developing a plan for yourself for the next several years.

It should, however, be candidly said that perhaps the most disturbing aspect of hormone replacement drugs is the assumption that the woman is deficient in female hormones. The reduction in female hormones is not a deficiency; it is a natural decrease in the body's ability to become pregnant. Assuming that this is a deficiency state is like assuming that a two-year-old girl is hormone-deficient because her breasts are not developed.

Some physicians assert that the more natural alternatives to hormone replacement therapy are unproven, and some even think that the alternatives are often strange bits of folklore that are closer to quackery than science. This perspective carries much irony since one of the most common hormone replacement drugs, Premarin, is actually taken from the urine of a pregnant horse.

Rather than call each other strange or weird, now more than ever it seems worthwhile for us to investigate systematically safe measures and to carefully evaluate when safer or more drastic measures can best be applied. Then, hopefully, "the change of life" can be a time for joy and personal transformation.

Here are some strategies to help the menopausal women maintain or reattain her zest. Also, see the Osteoporosis chapter for additional strategies, and depending upon the symptoms you experience, check out other chapters that describe your symptoms.

Don't dilate those blood vessels. Large meals, alcohol, coffee, spicy foods, and strong emotions can dilate blood vessels and cause the body to grow warmer. Don't add fuel to the fire of those hot flashes.

Fire extinguishers on hot flashes. Take 500–1,000 mg of vitamin C with each meal, as it strengthens capillaries and can help regulate body temperature. Vitamin C and vitamin B complex enhance the effectiveness of estrogen, thus helping the body adapt to the reduction of this hormone. Bioflavonoids work synergistically with vitamin C and should be taken with it. Taking 100–200 IUs of vitamin E and 50–100 mcg of selenium with meals helps the heart function and also helps the body regulate its temperature.

Replace the right hormones. Although most conventional physicians recommend using estrogen in hormone replacement therapy, a small but growing number of physicians are now saying that it is more important to replace progesterone than estrogen. By using a natural progesterone cream, you can often obtain relief of various symptoms of menopause and stimulate the body's natural production of estrogen.

Herbal extinguishers. The following herbal cocktail is great for women with hot flashes: black cohosh, licorice root, sarsaparilla, blessed thistle, false unicorn roots, red raspberry leaf, elder, and squaw vine. Mix a couple of tablespoons of this mixture and steep for 20 minutes. Drink a cup or two a day. Licorice root, elder, and unicorn roots contain a substance similar to estrogen, and sarsaparilla contains a substance similar to progesterone. If you have high blood pressure or water retention, don't use the licorice root.

An herb to pause the pause. Black cohosh may be the most researched herbal remedy for women during menopause. Studies have found that it reduces hot flashes, depression, and vaginal dryness. This research uses a standardized extract of one milligram of triterpenes per tablet. The recommended dose is two tablets twice a day.

A female ginseng. Dong quai is an herb that is considered a female ginseng. This tonifying herb is an overall body-strengthening remedy. It also contains folic acid and B$_{12}$, which helps prevent pernicious anemia.

Flower power. The Bach Flower Remedy called walnut flower is helpful for people during major changes in their lives. Place a couple of drops of it under the tongue as needed.

Bee yourself. Bee pollen contains both male and female hormones and can be effective in relieving hot flashes and other symptoms of menopause. Take a couple of bee pollen capsules twice a day, or at least 500 mg.

Those essential fatty acids. Essential fatty acids help protect your arteries and normalize your hormones. Sources of these good oils are tuna or salmon, as well as flaxseeds, borage seeds, and pumpkin seeds, all of which can be purchased in seed, powder, or oil form. Evening primrose oil is another good source of essential fatty acids. Take two or three capsules or one tablespoon of the oil two times a day with meals.

Go green. Spirulina and chlorella are algae that are nutrient-rich. They are such a good source of beta-carotene and various trace minerals that many people call them "super foods." Wheat, barley, and alfalfa grasses are also green super foods. Take them as directed on the label.

Fan the flames. Perhaps the simplest and quickest way to cool down during a hot flash is to pull out a small, battery-powered electric fan.

Douse the flames. By drinking lots of water, especially after exercising, you will help your body regulate its temperature.

Natural clothing. Natural-fiber clothing reduces some of the heat you feel during hot flashes.

How dry I am ... how dry I was. Vaginal dryness is a common symptom of menopausal women. Some simple lubricants can be used, including K-Y jelly, *Calendula* (marigold) cream, and coconut oil. You can also simply prick a vitamin E capsule and use a few drops of the oil. These various oils last longer than vegetable oils.

Consistent sex. This more-than-one-minute healing (hopefully!) helps to prevent vaginal dryness and swings in estrogen level. Research has shown that sexual desire does not decrease during menopause, and, in fact, it actually increases for many women.

The soy of menopause. Soybeans, peas, cucumbers and other legumes are rich in natural estrogens; eating them can help alleviate some symptoms of menopause. The

Japanese language doesn't have a term for *hot flashes;* perhaps this is because they eat so many soy products.

Are the side effects worth it? Estrogen-replacement drugs raise copper levels in the blood and lower zinc levels. Elevated copper can cause moodiness, and zinc deficiency can lead to depression. These symptoms are common problems of menopause, and estrogen drugs augment them. If you are feeling these emotions strongly and are taking these drugs, talk to your doctor. She or he may choose to lower your dose of estrogen or seek safer alternatives.

A *healthy dose of family and friends.* Research has found that women with restricted social networks (women with little family life and few friends) suffer the most serious symptoms of menopause. Take a dose of family and friends as much as possible.

You're not just getting older; you're evolving. The negative pictures of growing older can create additional wrinkles and worry warts, inside and out. Growing older is not the problem; it's the extra negative baggage carried with it that can weigh a person down. Be proud of surviving so long, and think of wrinkles as merit badges of survival.

May you die young ... as late in life as possible. Youth is a state of mind, not a specific age perimeter. Zest and love of life are ageless and create a radiance that can help deal with whatever difficulties you are experiencing during this transitional period in your life. If this zest is missing from your life, find it ... and enjoy yourself in this search!

24
nausea and vomiting

"To eat is human, to digest divine."
—MARK TWAIN

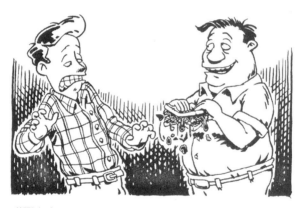

"This is a peanut butter sandwich with anchovies,
okra, and unripe pineapple in a garlic,
mustard, fudge sauce. I'm treating
nausea with my own homeopathic approach."

"Tossing cookies" sounds like a fun game, until you understand its slang meaning. While not an enjoyable activity, vomiting, throwing up, heaving, or whatever you prefer to call it is actually a valuable, even lifesaving defense of the body.

Gastric irritation can occur from ingesting poison or harmful bacteria, and nausea and vomiting are the body's forthright efforts to digest and eliminate this irritation in the quickest way possible. These processes are also the body's response to ingesting too much alcohol, too much food, or even just a little bit of a food that the body cannot efficiently digest. Nausea and vomiting are common for pregnant women during their first trimester. Despite the intense discomfort that morning sickness causes for pregnant women, the good news is that women who experience it also secrete higher amounts of hormones that actually reduce the chances of miscarriage or stillbirth. The body's efforts to protect itself are at work again.

The word *nausea* is actually derived from the Greek word for "ship." Nausea caused by seasickness and other forms of motion sickness seems to be an inherent response of the body to certain forms of disequilibrium.

Vomiting and nausea are also common for those who are stressed in a way that "makes you sick." Horror movies, disgusting sights, and cruel behavior can all lead to disequilibrium and gastric disturbances. Most people who feel nauseated have little or no appetite, which is another helpful defense of the body. So don't give any cookies to a person who tosses them! Here are some strategies to help you keep your cookies to yourself (also, see the chapter on Indigestion).

Don't add fuel to the fire. Try fasting, especially if you're not hungry. If you have an appetite, eat lightly, such as vegetable soup (the best choice), rice and steamed vegetables, toast, or grated apples. Avoid fats.

Liquidate yourself. Avoid dehydration from vomiting, especially if you have diarrhea at the same time. Drink vegetable broth, rice water (the excess water from cooking rice—this is great for nausea), carbonated water, or ginger ale. Drink in sips, not in gulps. Suck on ice chips if nothing else will stay down. Avoid coffee and black tea that can irritate your stomach.

Get cultured. Miso soup (made from fermented soy beans and/or other grains) can be made in a single minute and contains friendly bacteria that help you digest your food more efficiently. Yogurt also has these similar friendly bacteria; it's best to eat the plain, unflavored kind.

Take it gingerly. Ginger is a wonderfully effective remedy for nausea. Grate a tablespoon of fresh ginger root, and either make a tea with it or sprinkle it on applesauce.

Although fresh ginger will generally work best, there is evidence to show that simple powdered ginger is effective for nausea, including nausea caused by pregnancy. You can also consider adding in some anise seeds, either in whole form or those that are ground up.

Say hello to aloe. The juice from aloe vera is a great soothing and nourishing remedy for nausea. Drink ¼ cup upon rising, and another upon going to sleep.

Herbal aids. Make tea with either chamomile or peppermint, and drink it slowly and calmly. It will serve as a useful digestive aid.

Compress yourself. Apply hot compresses to the abdomen for three minutes, and then cold compresses for one minute. Repeat after 30 minutes.

Don't forget to breathe. Diaphragmatic breathing (as described in the Asthma section) is wonderfully relaxing and helps your body recharge itself.

Morning sickness vitamins. Some clinicians recommend taking up to 50 mg of vitamin B_6, 400 mg of magnesium, and 25 mg of zinc per day to combat nausea from pregnancy.

Ipecac for nausea? Ipecac is widely known as a substance that induces nausea and vomiting, and as a result, it is a common homeopathic medicine for treating such symptoms when given in very small doses. It is particularly helpful for people with acute persistent nausea who do not feel relieved after vomiting. They usually have little thirst and are nauseated by the smell of food. They often have increased salivation and a clean (not coated) tongue. *Ipecacuanha* 6 or 30 (ipecac in homeopathic doses) can be taken every other hour for a day.

Other little dabs to do ya. Another helpful homeopathic medicine is *Pulsatilla* (windflower). It is useful for people who experience nausea and/or vomiting after eating rich or fatty foods, especially ice cream. They tend to feel worse in warm rooms and feel better in a cool room. *Pulsatilla* 6 or 30 is recommended every three hours for a day. *Nux vomica* (poison nut) is commonly indicated for nausea or vomiting from mental exertion, after overeating, or from the use of alcohol, coffee, or drugs (therapeutic or recreational). It is for people who tend to be irritable and constipated. *Nux vomica* 6 or 30 is recommended every three hours for a day.

25

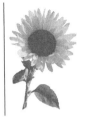

osteoporosis

"Loss is nothing else but change,
and change is Nature's delight."
—MARCUS AURELIUS

Both bones and eggshells are made primarily of calcium. Although bones can be impressively strong, depending upon their density, they can break like eggshells.

Osteoporosis, a common condition of the elderly, affects women more than men because they have less bone mass and because they produce less estrogen after menopause, which reduces the body's ability to keep calcium in the bones. Almost half of American women between 45 and 75 have some degree of osteoporosis. Osteoporosis is one of those silent diseases where the person doesn't experience any obvious symptoms until significant indicators, such as bone loss, have already occurred.

Osteoporosis leads to degeneration of the spine, which may result in humpback, and produces fragile bones that are more easily fractured. This condition is creating an elderly population that is fragile, weak, and, like an eggshell, breakable.

Osteoporosis is also creating a legion of shorter elderly people whose vertebrae are compressing against each other due to the loss of calcium from the bone. Perhaps this explains the origin of the Incredible Shrinking Woman's problem.

The epidemic of osteoporosis has created a major market for calcium supplementation. If calcium supplements were listed on the stock exchange, their price would have skyrocketed in recent years. However, if people knew about the following research about calcium, the stock's value would fall as fast as it rose.

There are numerous countries that have a very low rate of osteoporosis despite the fact that the people consume as little as 200 mg of calcium a day, considerably less than the 1,000–1,500 mg of calcium that most doctors recommend for pre- and postmenopausal women. The problem in this country is that most women consume too much of substances that leech the calcium out of the bones.

Research has shown that excessive protein, especially red meat (which contains 20 times more phosphorus than calcium), creates an imbalance in the body's calcium/phosphorus ratio, which is normally a little over 1:1. It has also been found that red meat stimulates release of parathyroid hormone, which promotes calcium excretion. Fats, especially saturated fats, also disrupt calcium absorption.

Eskimo women are known to have one of the highest rates of osteoporosis in the world, even though they eat more than 2,000 mg of calcium a day due to their consumption of fish bones and even though exercise is a regular part of their life. This problem is not due to bad luck. It is because they eat so much protein (as much as 250–400 grams a day) and so much fat that this excess causes increased calcium loss. This example highlights the importance of looking at factors that help *and* that hinder calcium absorption.

Conventional physicians often recommend hormone replacement therapy as a means to prevent osteoporosis. Research has shown that lifelong use of these hormones helps maintain bone strength, although it does not restore bone loss that has already occurred. More problematic regarding the use of these drugs are the numerous studies indicating their side effects, including increased chances of endometrial cancer and heart disease. Also, once a woman stops taking these drugs, calcium excretion is significantly increased.

Here are some strategies that are less costly than drugs, both financially and otherwise, and that have fewer side effects. Since having adequate calcium levels in the bone is dependent on building bone strength in the younger ages, it is best to do something about osteoporosis as early in life as possible. Although the best time to start was when you were a child, the second best time is today. Here are some strategies to stem bone loss and to turn it into bone gain.

Move your bod. Exercise, especially weight-bearing exercise such as walking, tennis, dancing, rope-jumping, basketball, and backpacking, helps build strong bones. Swimming is not considered a weight-bearing exercise because of the zero-gravity environment of water.

Do gentler, kinder exercises. Free the neck, power to the pelvis, liberate the vertebrae 31! Doing yoga and other gentle exercises helps make a person limber and stronger. However, people with osteoporosis should not do headstands and shoulderstands.

Calcium-rich foods. Sardines, salmon, green leafy vegetables, broccoli, tofu with calcium sulfate, mineral water, sesame seeds, milk, cheese, and yogurt all will supply your body with calcium.

Calcium blockers. Whole-grain foods contain certain chemicals that can impair calcium absorption. Avoid eating calcium-rich foods with whole grains in the same meal. Also, foods with oxalic acid can disrupt calcium assimilation; such foods include spinach, rhubarb, chard, chocolate, cashews, almonds, asparagus, and beet greens.

Avoid calcium vampires. "Calcium vampires" are substances that suck the calcium out of your bones. In other words, they stimulate the body to excrete more calcium than is being put into it. Substances that are calcium vampires are excessive protein (especially red meat), excessive fat, alcohol, caffeine, salt, tobacco, distilled water, and aluminum (absorbed from baking soda, aluminum pots, and from certain deodorants). Phosphorus-rich foods and drinks also impair calcium absorption, the worse offenders being soda drinks and many processed foods. Becoming aware of calcium vampires may be one of the most important strategies to prevent osteoporosis.

Avoid the calcium vampire drugs. Many drugs disrupt calcium absorption or metabolism, including antacids, antibiotics, antidepressants, anticonvulsants, anticoagulants, barbiturates, cholesterol-reducing drugs, corticosteroids, diuretics, laxatives, and chemotherapeutic drugs. Seek alternatives to these drugs, or expect their consequences.

Support stomach acid. An inadequate amount of stomach acid can lead to poor absorption of calcium. To increase stomach acid, eat charcoal (barbecued) foods or charcoal supplements, eat more slowly, and don't wash your food down too quickly with a drink. You might also consider taking a daily teaspoon of apple cider vinegar and/or the juice of a lemon in a cup of warm water.

Do the calcium-magnesium team. Calcium and magnesium are a duo that works together in your body, so if you take calcium, you should also take magnesium. Premenopausal women should take roughly 1,000 mg of calcium a day, and during menopause they should take about 1,500 mg. It is best to avoid taking large doses of calcium at one time; it is better to take smaller doses more frequently. Also, don't think that megadoses of calcium are better than the above recommendations; too much calcium can create problems because it displaces iron, manganese, and zinc, and it can lead to kidney stones. The dose of magnesium should be at least 50 percent of the dose of calcium. For additional help, take 1,000 mg of vitamin C, which helps to create collagenous fibers to which the calcium of the bone is attached.

Supplemental supplements. Boron, zinc, copper, and manganese are essential for bone integrity. They are all in green leafy vegetables. Boron is of special value; it has been found to stimulate higher estrogen levels and increase bone density. Supplementation of not more than 3 mg per day is recommended.

Go outside. Vitamin D is important for calcium absorption. You can ingest vitamin D by being exposed to the sun. Get a healthy dose of this sun vitamin (when possible, an hour or two per day), but don't overdo it.

Fish for fish oil. Fish oil has a healthy dose of vitamin D that helps the body absorb calcium.

Plant estrogens. Certain herbs are rich estrogens that are a significantly safer source of this important chemical than are hormone replacement drugs. These herbs also help balance estrogen levels in a woman so that they can actually help reduce estrogen levels if they are too high and augment them if they are too low. Some good sources of plant estrogens are black cohosh, dong quai, liquorice, unicorn root, and fennel. Herbal formulas with one or more of these herbs in pill or extract form are readily available in health food stores and pharmacies.

Horsetail tea. It won't grow you a tail, but this herb is rich in calcium and silica and can help build strong bones. Consider drinking a cup a day for a week, stop doing it for a week, start again for a week, and repeat.

Be born black. While this is not a one-minute strategy, evidence does show that black people do not experience as much osteoporosis as white people do, possibly because they have greater bone mass.

26

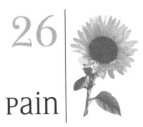

pain

> *"The great engineer of the universe has made man as perfectly as he could make him, and he could not have invented a better device for his maintenance than to provide him with a sense of pain."*
>
> —RENÉ DESCARTES

Pain has been referred to as a temporary condition caused by a deficiency of morphine. As preposterous as this may sound, this statement actually isn't too far from the truth, for the body does create its own opiate-like substances called endorphins that deaden pain. Even Nancy Reagan wouldn't "say no" to these internal drugs. Luckily, you can't get arrested for carrying opiate derivatives in your brain.

Pain is a very subjective feeling. The International Association for the Study of Pain defines *pain* as an unpleasant sensory or emotional experience associated with actual or potential tissue damage. Whatever the source or nature of the pain, it is calling, even demanding, your attention. Pain is an inherent protective device that nature has given us. It is sometimes difficult to acknowledge the value of pain while one is experiencing its wrath. Still, pain is absolutely essential for the survival of the human species. Among other benefits, it encourages us to learn from our mistakes and to avoid potentially dangerous experiences. Seeking to understand what it is saying is worthwhile, though not always easy.

The most common chronic pain syndromes are backache, headache, joint pain, and pain from injury. Pain itself is not a disease, but is a symptom of disease or injury. Simply treating the pain doesn't necessarily change the condition, and this is why painkillers offer only short-term relief at best.

Conventional medical treatment for pain usually consists of medication, nerve blocks, and surgery. Although these approaches may provide certain benefits, they encourage you to be passive, giving you a sense that you don't have much control over your own pain or your own life.

The following strategies will help you take greater control of your pain and hopefully eradicate it or at least reduce it to more manageable levels. These strategies will help you manage your pain before it manages you.

Breathe into the pain. Resisting pain can sometimes aggravate it, just like trying to untie a knot by pulling at both ends. Taking a deep abdominal breath into and through the pain can be relaxing and healing. Focus your attention on the pain, and imagine you are inhaling and exhaling through the primary site of pain. Breathing into the pain while doing yoga exercises can provide additional therapeutic effects.

Get in hot water. Sitting in a hot bath can be wonderfully restorative.

Get tense. Tightening the area around the pain for a couple of seconds and then releasing it is a good trick to reduce the pain.

Get to the point. There are acupressure points all over your body that can effectively reduce the pain and start the healing. The best points are never precisely on the primary place of pain. Seek out "trigger points"—that is, points that seem hypersensitive to the touch. Sometimes suitable points are around joints that are near the pain, and sometimes they are on the other side of the body parallel to where the pain is. Press the point firmly with your thumb for five seconds, release, and then repeat the pressure several times.

Get it handed to you. Ask a friend to practice the laying on of hands, which is an ancient healing practice that is used today by thousands of nurses and other health professionals in hospitals. The person doing it should concentrate, and imagine loving and healing energies emitting from his or her hands into your body. Your friend may choose to hold his or her hands near the area of pain, although you should encourage your friend to use intuition to determine where to apply the energy. While your friend is there, perhaps he or she can also give you a massage, which can be wonderfully relaxing and pain relieving.

Have a spicy life. Eat chili peppers. They contain capsaicin that has been found to stimulate secretion of endorphins and reduce the release of a neurotransmitter, substance P, which short-circuits the perception of pain. There are also external ointments sold in health food stores and pharmacies that contain capsaicin.

Coffee for pain relief. There is a good reason why most aspirin tablets contain caffeine: It can block opiate receptors in the brain and reduce the sensation of pain. Although coffee may provide this beneficial effect, don't fool yourself into thinking that it is "curing" you. It isn't, but it is providing temporary relief while you figure out deeper healing strategies.

Reduce your ingestion of animal fat. At first blush, this strategy may seem odd and questionably useful. However, the inflammatory process is a part of many pain syndromes, and animal fat is the only source of arachidonic acid, an important precursor to prostaglandins that can augment inflammation. By reducing your intake of animal fat, you can reduce some inflammation.

Dear diary. Keep a pain journal. By observing carefully when and where you experience pain, you can sometimes find certain patterns to it, and then try to break or change these patterns. You may, for instance, discover that you develop your symptoms when you don't get enough sleep, don't get adequate physical exercise, miss a meal, eat certain foods, or visit relatives. Perhaps a surgical procedure called relative-ectomy may be indicated.

Describe and draw the pain. Describe the pain in as much detail as possible, and then draw it with crayons or colored pens or pencils. Imagine and draw the shapes and colors that you feel may soothe the pain; visualize these colors and shapes in your body.

Mental technology. Research on biofeedback has not only shown its value in teaching people to relax, but it has shown that it can also influence many bodily functions. Biofeedback is very valuable for teaching people to have greater control and direction over their bodies, and thus, over their pain.

Meditation technology. Meditation not only helps people achieve a greater state of relaxation, it encourages more focused concentration, giving you better control of your mind as well as greater control over your sense of pain.

Hypnotize yourself. Autohypnosis is a popular technique for relaxation and can be used effectively for healing and pain control. One hypnosis strategy, called glove anesthesia, is to put yourself in a trance and imagine your hand to be numb, heavy, and wooden. Then, move your hand to the part or parts of the body that feel pain, and imagine that those parts are feeling similarly relaxed, heavy, and numb.

Exercise and exorcise the demons out. Research has found that exercise increases endorphin levels in the blood. The increase in these opiate-like substances is one reason that athletes sometimes feel "high" when they are exercising. Likewise, exercise may help reduce your pain. However, this strategy should not be considered if exercise induces pain.

Massage the sole. Your feet, especially the bottoms, have thousands of nerve endings, and by massaging them, you are stimulating various parts of the body that the nerves feed, thus reducing pain. The joy and relaxation that massaging the feet creates is good for the sole and the soul.

Smell your pain away. The essential oils of lavender and chamomile have relaxing and sedating properties that can provide pain relief. Consider soaking in a bath in which a couple of drops from the essential oils of these flowers are added, or simply place some drops on a handkerchief and sniff your troubles away.

Believe in belief. Whatever you do to relieve your pain, believe in it and it will work better. Research has shown that approximately 33 percent of people with pain experience relief of symptoms from a placebo.

Distract yourself. Try not to let pain interfere with your life. Keep busy with activities that require concentration so that you can forget about your pain for a while.

Misery loves company. Consider joining a support group of people who experience chronic pain. It's best to avoid groups that simply complain about their problems; instead, seek out one that shares information about strategies that are helpful in dealing with pain.

Empower yourself. A sense of control over one's life is therapeutic in itself. The decision to try some strategies to help yourself may be almost as helpful as ultimately doing them.

27
premenstrual syndrome (PMS)

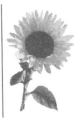

"Nothing in our society, with the exception of violence and fear, has been more effective in keeping women in their place than the degradation of the menstrual cycle."
— CHRISTIANE NORTHRUP, M.D.

Various cycles and rhythms permeate nature. The rise and fall of the sun, the evolution of the seasons, and the ebb and flow of the tides are mirrored in our bodies: our waking and sleeping cycle; the spring, summer, fall, and autumn of our lives; and the rhythmic flow of our blood. Despite our acceptance of these cycles and rhythms, Western civilization has not granted the same dignity and honor to women's monthly cycle of menstruation. It is generally viewed as a chore, an indignity, or at least something that one should not discuss.

Is it any wonder that the shadow that we helped to create comes back to haunt us?

During a typical menstrual cycle, a woman produces between two and four ounces of blood. A single super-absorbent tampon is able to soak up one or more ounces of fluid, which is usually considerably more than a woman's vagina creates during the time it is inserted. This tampon also soaks up other vaginal secretions that are vital for the healthy function of a woman's reproductive organs, leading to vaginal ulceration, lesions, lacerations, and sometimes infections. This situation not only can result in cases of potentially fatal Toxic Shock Syndrome, it much more frequently leads to immune system disruptions, including autoimmune diseases.

Approximately 50 percent of all women experience various physical and/or psychological symptoms prior to their menstruation. Some of them experience quite mild symptoms, while others can have reactions dramatic enough to turn Dr. Jekyll into Ms. Hyde.

In the not-too-distant past, physicians commonly believed that the various troubles that women claimed to experience prior to their menstruation were all in their head. It is a relief that physicians finally recognize a physiological component to premenstrual syndrome, although simply recognizing a condition as valid is not enough to cure it.

Some physicians theorize that PMS results from a drop in progesterone, sometimes called the "tranquility hormone." Others think that soaring estrogen levels lead to irritable and anxious states. Still others believe that the body's awareness that conception did not occur depresses women physically and psychologically. Whatever the cause, women commonly experience a variety of symptoms from the biological warfare occurring in their body, including cramps, breast swelling and tenderness, water retention, moodiness, irritability, headaches, backaches, insomnia, fatigue, constipation, complexion problems, and food cravings.

The premenstrual state, however, does offer some positive effects. Many women experience a greater ability to concentrate, more creativity, and more assertiveness during this period. It is a time to clean and organize their home and life. Some women who feel more emotional during this special time cherish these feelings and honor them as an integral part of who they are.

A woman friend celebrates her altered state by wearing some special jewelry during her premenstrual period. This one-minute strategy helps her, her partner, and friends become aware of this more sensitive phase of the month so that Dr. Jekyll and Ms. Hyde are more self-conscious, empathetic, and friendly to each other.

And here are some more strategies.

A low-fat diet reduces weight and PMS. Several studies have indicated that women who eat a low-fat diet have less breast swelling and fewer of the other uncomfortable symptoms during their premenstrual period.

Exercise, and leave PMS in the dust. Regular exercise has been found to reduce PMS. Besides increasing the brain's secretion of natural painkilling endorphins, exercise helps to tonify and relax muscles, improve circulation, and reduce water retention.

Avoid the PMS aggravators. The following substances can aggravate PMS: coffee (even the decaffeinated variety), black tea, chocolate, colas, salt, dairy products, fats, and alcohol.

Keep track of yourself. Keep a diary and watch for habits or patterns in your life that seem to aggravate your condition. You may discover that certain foods, stresses, emotional states, birth control pill dosages, or levels of exercise aggravate or ameliorate your symptoms.

Every body does not need milk. Experiment by eliminating milk and milk products from your diet. Some women are allergic to them, and for others the increased calcium may disrupt the calcium-magnesium balance in the body, leading to cramps and heavy periods.

Oil yourself. Evening primrose oil and other oils (flaxseed, borage, black currant seed, and pumpkin seed) are excellent sources of essential fatty acids, which play an essential role in creating a natural hormone called prostoglandins, which can relieve premenstrual symptoms. It is recommended to take 200 mg of evening primrose oil for the ten days preceding your menstrual flow. Consider using these oils in your recipes instead of other types of oils, especially when making salad dressings and other unheated recipes.

Supplementary, my dear Ms. Watson. About two days before you expect to begin your PMS time, take calcium up to 1,500 mg, magnesium up to 1,000 mg, vitamin A up to 10,000 IU, vitamin D up to 400 IU, and B complex (especially B$_6$) with 50–100 mg of the major components. The B vitamins have calming effects on a woman's emotional state, calcium is important for reducing cramps, and several of the other vitamins help the body absorb and make use of it. Remember, do not take large doses of these vitamins all at once; the body is best able to absorb smaller doses taken more frequently, and preferably with meals.

Don't cramp your style. Here are some great herbs to reduce the pain and discomfort of menstrual cramps: black cohosh root, false unicorn root, squaw vine, blessed thistle, lobelia, pennyroyal, and red raspberry. This combination of herbs doesn't taste great, but wouldn't you rather drink something that doesn't *taste* good than cramps that don't make you *feel* good? Drink a couple of cups of this tea throughout the day. A more simplified version of this concoction is black cohosh root and red raspberry. For those who wish to avoid bad-tasting tea, blend these herbs into a powder and encapsulate them. Take one to three caps a day, as needed, and don't drink any caffeinated beverages the same day.

More herbs to de-cramp your style. Chamomile and peppermint are both wonderfully soothing herbs that reduce cramping and improve digestion. Make a tea of one or the other, for they work best when they are not combined.

Yam it up. Wild yam cream contains a natural form of progesterone that some women have found effective in relieving PMS. The cream can be rubbed onto the chest, inner arms, thighs, and abdomen soon after ovulation. Wild yam extract is also useful when ingested in pill form.

Yogis don't get PMS. Or, at least, they don't get it very badly. A survey of 848 women who practice yoga showed that 77 percent of them experienced reduced symptoms of PMS after practicing yoga. The corpse pose is great for relaxing and is best done during the early stages of PMS. This pose looks just like it sounds: Lay flat on your back with your legs and arms slightly spread, melt into the floor, and feel relaxation spread over your body. Another good yogic posture is the forward bend, which can be done by sitting on the floor with legs together straight out in front of you and bending your upper torso so that you can touch your toes—or at least your ankles. Try to hold the forward bend as long as you can do so comfortably, and continue to breathe slowly and deeply.

The hot and cold treatment. Hot and cold packs to the abdominal area and lower back can be helpful. The hot application should be used for three minutes, and the cold application for one minute. Repeat this two to four times.

Hot stuff. Take a hot bath, drink hot tea, and apply a hot pad to your abdomen (but not necessarily all at the same time).

Super acupressure. This acupressure treatment for relieving menstrual or premenstrual cramps doesn't use your thumbs, but rather your fists. Place them on your lower back while you lie down. To help you apply firmer pressure, lie on your back on the floor with your feet on a chair or couch. You can also use tennis balls.

Get touched. Ask a friend or spouse to massage your back, abdomen, head, neck, and anywhere that it feels good to do so. Massage will not only relax you, but will also help you feel better.

*A **sexy strategy.*** Have sex. It is uncertain if orgasms have a direct effect on relieving cramps or if they simply take your mind off the pain . . . but who cares as long it works? Don't limit this method to a one-minute strategy.

*A **Sleep on it.*** Get plenty of sleep. It not only relaxes, but invigorates you, too.

*A **Homeopathic relief.*** *Magnesia phosphorica* (phosphate of magnesium) is indicated when warmth and doubling up relieve menstrual cramps. *Colocynthis* (bitter cucumber) is helpful when the menstrual pains almost force you to double up and when you're feeling a heightened state of irritability. *Chamomilla* (chamomile) is useful for the most severe, unbearable cramping pains and when you're extremely irritable. Whatever medicine fits your symptoms, take it in the 6 or 30 potency every three hours during the discomfort. Stop taking the remedy if the pain stops or if there isn't obvious relief after 48 hours.

*A **dab for the emotions, too.*** Homeopathic doses of *Pulsatilla* and *Ignatia* are wonderfully effective for the emotional swings of PMS. *Pulsatilla* 6 or 30 is particularly helpful for the weepy, moody, and self-pitying PMS woman; while *Ignatia* 6 or 30 is indicated for the irritable, misunderstood, and brooding PMS woman.

Get pregnant. This strategy is only temporarily effective and has its own side effects.

Get pregnant II. New research indicates that women who have had a child experience less pain during their menstrual cycle than women who have never given birth.

28 sinusitis

"When the head aches, all the members feel the pain."
—FROM *DON QUIXOTE,* BY CERVANTES

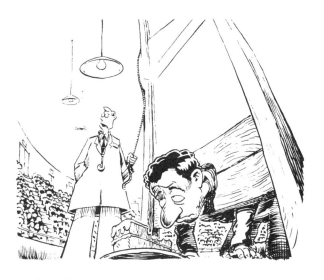

A professor at the Marie Antoinette School
of Medicine teaches the proper treatment
for sinusitis.

The next time someone tells you that you have a hole in your head, simply admit that you do. We all do. In fact, there are eight holes in the skull. Commonly called sinuses, these cavities play an important role in respiration. If we didn't have cavities, just solid bone, our neck probably couldn't support the weight of this top-heavy condition, thus causing us to hang our head in evolutionary shame.

Inflammation in these sinuses, called sinusitis, creates head pain, facial tenderness, eyeball aching, and even a sensation that feels like the teeth are long. These symptoms make sinusitis sound like a type of torture, as any sufferer will confirm.

Sinusitis is most often the revenge of a lingering cold or allergy, which can impede proper nasal drainage. This congestion becomes a breeding ground for infection that then leads the lining in the sinuses to become inflamed and swollen. Other problems that can create congestion leading to sinusitis are polyps, a deviated septum, large or inflamed adenoids, an abscessed or inflamed tooth, or a change in air pressure from flying or swimming.

Sinusitis can create its own revenge, too. Unless it is successfully treated, it can sometimes lead to ear infection, pneumonia, or bronchitis.

Although sinusitis sufferers may want to hire Roto-Rooter to unplug their nose and drain their head, these other strategies should be considered first.

A saltwater nasal spray. Perhaps the best nasal spray (and the cheapest!) is salt and water. Place ¼ teaspoon of salt and four ounces of water in a squirt gun or spray bottle, and shoot yourself in the nose with it. The salt and water combined will help break up nasal congestion. Blow your nose gently afterwards.

Get steamed. Inhaling steam can feel great. Either drape a towel over your head and stand over a pot of boiling water, or take a hot steam shower. For a little added therapeutic action, add eucalyptus leaves or eucalyptus oil to the boiling water.

Get hot and cold. Alternate hot and cold compresses and place them over the cheekbones and nostrils. Tip your head slightly forward to encourage better drainage through the nose.

Impress yourself. Firm pressure in a circular motion on acupressure points under the eyebrows, on the cheekbones, and at the base of each nostril can work wonders.

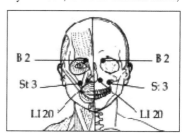

The massage is the message. Massaging the neck, shoulders, and skull may or may not cure you, but it will feel great. Because there are so many nerve endings in your feet, especially on the bottoms, massaging them can sometimes soothe the nervous system and be relaxing to the entire body. According to the foot massage system of reflexology, massaging the big toe can be particularly helpful to people with sinusitis.

Jog it out of you. Jogging and other vigorous exercise can help drain sinuses.

Just say no to alcohol. Alcohol causes increased vasodilation, which means that the blood vessels swell and lead to more congestion and inflammation.

Head to the ocean. Swimming in or even being near the ocean offers relief to many sinusitis sufferers. Avoid being in valleys, because pollen tends to live there and can aggravate this condition.

Don't get smoked. Exposure to cigarette smoke, even secondhand smoke, can be very irritating to the sinuses. Some people will be irritated by a barbecue or by smog. Avoid these irritants whenever possible.

Drink up. Drink lots of fluids (except alcohol) to keep the mucus flowing.

Chicken soup to the rescue, again. Hot chicken soup has been found to stimulate mucus drainage.

Don't blow your brains out. When you blow your nose, do it gently. Blowing too strongly can force the infected mucus back into the sinuses. If blowing your nose sounds like a wildlife mating call, you are blowing too hard.

A sound idea. Making a repetitious sound sometimes provides relief. Experiment with various sounds such as "ahhhhhh," "eeeeee," "ommmmmm," or whatever other sound works for you. Additional benefits are possible if you close your eyes and relax while you say these sounds.

Avoid dry heat. If the heating system in your house or office is providing heat that is too dry, use a humidifier to moisten the air. Check the humidifier regularly for the growth of mold or mildew. If an air conditioner is used, make certain its filter is kept clean.

Spice up your life. Chili peppers, garlic, and horseradish encourage mucus secretion. Add them to meals whenever possible, or simply take capsules of them.

Chop an onion. Chopping onions will trigger crying and a loosening of mucus in the head that may make it easier for you to expel it and clear your head.

Don't pull the triggers. Because sinusitis can be precipitated by a food allergy, it is recommended to avoid (at least temporarily) the most common food allergy triggers: milk, wheat, corn, citrus, eggs, and peanut butter.

Seal up those sinuses. Goldenseal is the most important herbal medicine for bacterial sinus infections. Take the fluid extract, freeze-dried root, or powdered solid extract at least every two hours. Be warned, however, that goldenseal is a bitter-tasting herb (it is very medicinal tasting). Don't take it for longer than a week at a time, and don't take it at all if you're pregnant.

Avoid antihistamines. Although these drugs reduce nasal swelling, they also dry the mucous membranes and therefore encourage greater congestion. It is better to use strategies that stimulate drainage than stifle it.

Avoid decongestants. Decongestants paralyze the nose hairs (the cilia), thus inhibiting the drainage of fluids. They also cause "rebound congestion," a temporary relief of congestion only to be followed by an increase in it. People also develop a tolerance to this drug and need stronger and stronger doses of it for it to be effective. Avoid nasal sprays, too.

Don't chlorinate your nose. If you swim, wear a nose plug to prevent chlorinated water from further irritating the sinuses.

Stay grounded. If possible, avoid flying or engaging in activities that take you to high altitudes that can be aggravating to a sinus condition.

Homeopathic help. *Kali bic* 6 or 30 (also called *Kali bichromicum*) is an effective homeopathic medicine for sinus pain at the root of the nose, especially when the person's nasal discharge is thick and stringy. *Pulsatilla* 6 or 30 is more commonly given to women or children with sinus problems, especially when their symptoms are worse at night, in a warm room, or when stooping. People who need *Pulsatilla* may have digestive symptoms that accompany the sinus pains. If you don't know how to individualize a homeopathic medicine for your unique sinusitis symptoms, you might consider trying one of the sinusitis products that contain several different homeopathic medicines. Take a dose every four hours if you have mild pain, and every two hours during intense pain. If you don't feel better within 24 hours, consider another strategy.

29

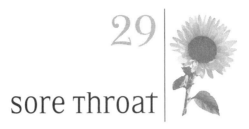

sore throat

"Get the facts first. You can distort them later."
—MARK TWAIN

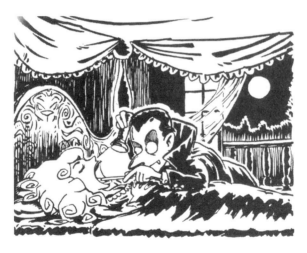

A little-known fact: Health-conscious Dracula tests
his victims for strep throat before biting them.

The throat takes a lot of abuse. It is subjected to bacterial and viral infection; to various airborne irritants such as dust, smoke, and fumes; and to vocal use (and use and use). Considering all the food that we shove down our throat, often with minimal chewing, it's amazing that our throat doesn't figuratively *grab* us by the throat, and it's amazing that it still speaks to us.

Like so many other parts of the body, the throat is quite durable. And yet, it does have its limits. If necessary, it leaves us speechless or chokes us up with emotion. It gives us a lump in the throat or a pain in the neck. It will be rough to us or will make it difficult for us to swallow all these cliches.

Viruses and bacteria can cause a sore throat, but so can open-mouth breathing, artificially heated air, vocal overuse, and anything that creates a dry throat. More than 90 percent of sore throats in adults are viral, for which antibiotics are not recommended. Streptococcus is the most common bacteria to cause a sore throat. Most physicians recommend taking an antibiotic for such infections— not necessarily for the throat pain, but primarily to prevent the possibility of rheumatic fever, a life-threatening condition that is thought to result from the strep traveling to and infecting the heart.

The commonly held assumption that links strep throat to rheumatic fever, however, may not be accurate. According to a recent study, 33 to 50 percent of children with rheumatic fever develop it without having sore throat symptoms. And in a recent epidemic of rheumatic fever among children in Utah, two-thirds had no clear history of a sore throat within three months of the onset of rheumatic fever. More startling is that eight of the eleven children who tested positive for strep and who were prescribed antibiotics still developed rheumatic fever. This evidence suggests that it is questionable if sore throats are related to rheumatic fever, and even if they are, antibiotics do not seem to prevent this condition anyway.

Because the throat plays such an important role in our lives, here are some strategies to make certain that it stays in working order and still talks to us.

Gargle treatment #1. The combination of salt and water is a classic gargle treatment. Just mix about ¼ teaspoon of salt with ¼ cup of water, and gargle. Use this and the following other gargles as often as you feel it is necessary and helpful.

Gargle treatment #2. Sage or mullein tea is often healing to sore throats. Steep one teaspoon of the herb in a cup of water. Gargle for at least ten seconds with three different mouthfuls of tea.

Gargle treatment #3. Place five to ten drops of the tincture of myrrh into a cup of warm water, and gargle with it.

Since Biblical times, people have used myrrh, and it is known today to have antiseptic and astringent effects.

Gargle treatment #4. Take the leftover water from cooked barley, and add lemon to it for this helpful, soothing gargle.

Gargle treatment #5. For stubborn sore throats, take a cotton swab and thoroughly coat the back of the throat with the oil of bitter orange. Expect to gag a bit from this, but it can be worth it.

Herbal antibiotics. Echinacea and goldenseal are probably the most effective herbs for treating infections, so if your sore throat is the result of infection rather than from throat irritation, one or more of these herbs should be used. It is best to use echinacea in a fluid extract form. Numerous herbal formulas include echinacea and goldenseal together. Take ½ teaspoon three times a day.

An herbal soother. Slippery elm tablets are an old tried-and-true remedy for sore throat. Their soothing qualities protect mucous membranes in a dry and burning throat. People who can withstand the funny taste and strange consistency of slippery elm bark tea should make a brew. You can help improve the taste by adding some honey and fresh lemon.

Scare it out of you. Garlic has some powerful antiviral effects. Consider cutting up two fresh cloves of garlic and placing it some vegetable juice or chicken broth. If you are less brave, take garlic capsules three times a day.

Vaporize yourself. Steam inhalation can be helpful, especially if you add herbs such as sage, thyme, and/or mullein to the water. Stand over this boiling brew with a towel over your head.

A vitamin C lozenge. A 500 mg tablet of vitamin C should be slowly sucked so that its acidic nature can burn out the infection.

Zinc lozenges. Zinc lozenges are also effective in treating sore throats and colds. However, it is not recommended to take them regularly—only to prevent or treat a sore throat or cold—and don't take more than 150 mg a day.

Make room for mushrooms. Maitake, shiitake, and reishi mushrooms stimulate immune response and help fight viral infection. Take them as directed on the label.

First-stage homeopathics. *Aconitum* (monkshood) 6 or 30 is recommended for the first stage of a throat infection. It is particularly good when you have a dry throat and dry cough, especially if you have developed it after exposure to cold, dry winds. Take it every other hour for a day. If your symptoms do not abate after a single night's rest, consider another homeopathic medicine or strategy.

Bee venom homeopathics. If you have the type of sore throat where there is burning or stinging pain with much swelling, relieved by sucking on an ice cube or drinking cold fluids, take *Apis* (crushed bee) 6 or 30. Because bee venom is known to cause these burning and stinging pains, homeopathic doses of bee venom can initiate a healing response of these pains. Take it three to six times a day, depending on the intensity of the symptoms. You should not have to take it more than two days, or it isn't the correct medicine.

For those scarlet throats. If your symptoms include scarlet-red tonsils, a reddened face and lips, and a fever, then *Belladonna* (deadly nightshade) 6 or 30 is the homeopathic medicine for you. Take it three to six times a day, depending on the intensity of your discomfort. If it doesn't work within 48 hours, consider another strategy.

That fishbone feeling. If you have one of those sore throats that feels like a fishbone or stick is caught in it, consider taking *Hepar sulphur* (calcium sulphide) 6 or 30. This homeopathic medicine is particularly effective when you are relieved by warm drinks and irritated by cold ones and tend to be chilly and easily aggravated by cold air.

Drugs can dry you out. Various prescription and over-the-counter drugs can dry out your throat and then lead to laryngitis or a sore throat. Check with your doctor to determine if your drugs should be changed or reduced.

Throw your toothbrush away! Although I know you may think this is a totally useless strategy, be aware that using and reusing an old toothbrush may reinfect you. Researchers have estimated that toothbrushes carry more than a million bacteria. A thorough rinsing of the brush is thought to reduce this number by only one half, so it may be prudent to throw away a toothbrush after throat and respiratory infections, and to replace it regularly—at least every three months.

The anti-antibiotic things. If you are on antibiotics, there are certain common mineral supplements and foods that can inhibit their action. Mineral supplements such as iron, calcium, magnesium, and zinc can inactivate certain antibiotics (including tetracycline, ciprofloxacin, and norfloxacin). Also, grapefruit juice can actually help expel the antibiotic from the bloodstream, rendering it ineffective.

30

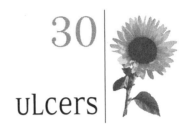

ulcers

There once was an ulcer from Ulster,
'Twas in a youngster, not oldster,
From stress it arose,
At times it dozed,
That ulcer had a mind of its ownster.

The average adult has 35 million digestive glands. These glands produce one of the most powerful corrosives known—gastric acid. Gastric acid is so strong that it can dissolve a razor blade in less than a week. As a result, the body must create a new stomach lining every three days.

Actually, stomach acid isn't "the bad guy." Stomach acid is not only essential for digesting foods, it is vital for our survival because it kills fungi, bacteria, and viruses that are ingested with food. If we didn't have the protection that the gastric acid gives us, we would be more susceptible to food poisoning, parasites, and other digestive dilemmas—including ulcers.

Research has now confirmed that most people with

ulcers actually have a normal amount of gastric acid. The problem isn't having too much acid; it's in the body's ability to keep the lining of the stomach intact.

The initial symptoms of an ulcer are usually belching and bloating, which can mislead the sufferer into thinking that you are just experiencing gas. You may also feel hunger pangs and a burning, gnawing, and/or sharp pain in the abdominal area. The pains tend to be felt 45 to 60 minutes after eating a meal, although they can also be experienced on an empty stomach. The pains tend to be temporarily relieved by eating food. Because ulcers can create medical emergencies, people with an ulcer, or those who think that they may have one, should seek medical attention.

Relatively recently, researchers discovered that a type of bacteria, *Helicobacter pylori,* may cause ulcers. Antibiotics have become the treatment of choice because of this assumption. However, antibiotics can aggravate digestive problems and create new ones.

Not too long ago, the most common advice that doctors gave ulcer patients was to eat a bland diet: usually boiled fish, rice, steamed vegetables, and milk; no spices, pizza, or chili; and no Mexican, Italian, Indian, or Thai food (bummer!). As it turns out, this wasn't such good advice, as there is no real evidence that spicy foods cause or exacerbate ulcers (whew!).

There are, however, certain foods, drinks, and behaviors

that can increase gastric acids and thus create a problem for those people who are not adequately replacing their stomach lining every three days. Here are some ulcer do's and don'ts.

Milk burns! Although milk initially coats the stomach walls, providing temporary relief, the stomach secretes increased acid to digest the milk, ultimately making stomach discomforts worse than before. Avoid this rebound effect by avoiding milk.

Painkillers can be stomach killers. Aspirin is known to cause increased bleeding in the stomach that can exacerbate an ulcer. By the way, some antacids, notably Alka-Seltzer, contain aspirin, so be careful of what antacid you take. Even worse than aspirin are nonsteroidal anti-inflammatory drugs such as Motrin or Advil that can irritate the stomach lining and aggravate an ulcer.

Eat smaller meals. Eating smaller meals more frequently is less stressful on your digestive system than eating two or three larger meals. Chew every bite thoroughly.

Pump iron, but don't ingest it. Don't take iron supplements; they can irritate the stomach. There are, however, exceptions to this general rule: In some people with ulcers who lose a lot of blood, they may become anemic and need iron. Even then, rather than taking iron supplements as a first resort, there are easier, healthier ways to add iron to your diet (see the chapter on Anemia for details).

Supplement your stomach lining. Vitamins A, B_6, E, and folic acid help maintain and repair the stomach lining. Zinc can also be helpful.

Ulcer accomplices. Smoking, alcohol, and caffeine don't "cause" ulcers, but they do reduce the stomach's ability to protect itself, thus increasing the chances that you'll get an ulcer.

An ulcer's friends. Fried foods, citrus fruits, chocolate, alcohol, black tea, and coffee (regular and decaffeinated) increase gastric acids and can aggravate your ulcer.

Fiberize. Fiber can be helpful because it helps to coat and soothe the stomach lining, but avoid foods that have abrasive roughage, such as nuts, seeds, and popcorn. Grains, legumes, fruits, and vegetables are great sources of fiber. Oat bran and wheat bran can be particularly good as well.

A cabbage patch will patch your stomach. Cabbage juice is high in L-glutamine, an amino acid that stimulates the secretion of mucus from the stomach's lining. More than just a folk medicine, cabbage juice has been proven to be effective in treating ulcers. Drink juice only from fresh green cabbages. If they are unavailable where you are, you can use celery juice, which also has ulcer-healing compounds.

Is that a banana in your pocket? Unripe plantain bananas, an old folk remedy for ulcers, can now be obtained in a dried extract, pill-form. These bananas contain a substance that is known to stimulate mucus from the stomach lining, providing a sturdier barrier against gastric acids.

Lick an ulcer with licorice root. Licorice root has been used for centuries in herbal medicine for various conditions, including ulcers. Its protective effects on the stomach lining reduce stomach discomfort. You can obtain a piece of the root from an herb or health food store; it is recommended to suck on it for 20 minutes before meals. For people who aren't "suckers," you can obtain licorice root in tablet or capsule form. People with high blood pressure must be careful with this herb because it can elevate blood pressure. Such individuals should take a new product, deglycyrrhizinated licorice, which eliminates this potential problem; it is available in health food stores.

A slippery soother. Slippery elm is one of the most effective herbs in botanical medicine for soothing inflamed mucous membranes or ulcers. Simply pour boiling water over slippery elm powder and let it steep for ten minutes. Make certain to stir occasionally so that a "Nestle's Quick Effect" (the settling of the powder to the bottom of the glass) does not occur. Sip.

An Indian spice is nice. Turmeric, a popular Indian spice, has been found to protect the stomach lining due to its powerful antioxidant effects. Consider adding it to whatever food you cook, but expect its yellow-orangish nature to turn your food this color.

An ulcer extinguisher. Aloe vera is known to be very effective in treating burns and can likewise put out the fire of an ulcer. If you have a fresh aloe plant, open one of the stalks of the plant and spoon out the watery gel, and blend it with water and drink it. If you don't have a plant, get aloe vera juice from a health food store. (Make certain that the juice you purchase is digestible; health food stores sell many inedible cosmetics made with aloe vera.)

The seaweed treatment. Nori, the type of seaweed in which sushi is usually wrapped, has an anti-ulcer substance in it. It also has antimicrobial action against many disease-causing bacteria. You can eat it with sushi; or simply take the sheets of nori, dampen and cut them, and add it to salads, steamed vegetables, or grain dishes.

Take two breaths, and call me in the morning. Relax, take a couple of deep breaths, relax more deeply, take a couple more deep breaths, and relax more deeply.

De-stress yourself. Although there is presently insufficient evidence to show that stress causes ulcers, it is known that if you already have an ulcer, stress can worsen it. Actually, it isn't the stress that's the problem; it's our response to the stress that can aggravate an ulcer. Do whatever is necessary to both reduce the amount of stress you are experiencing and to learn to deal with whatever stress you *do* experience.

Slow down. Walk and drive more slowly, eat and drink more slowly, and respond to phone calls and doorbells more slowly. You'll still get there, feel better, and may even enjoy everything a little bit more.

Express yourself. Pent-up feelings, especially anger, can irritate you psychologically and physically. Express whatever you are feeling. If your feelings cannot be expressed in words, go to a place where you won't disturb others, and scream. Screaming in your car or into a pillow are probably the two most common ways to release your frustrations.

31

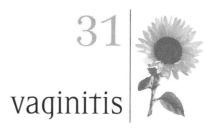

vaginitis

S cratching an itch is one of life's great pleasures, but not every itch can be scratched, especially in public. When this itching also burns and is accompanied by a discharge, you have an even greater problem. Such is the situation with vaginitis.

It is no surprise that the vagina is a perfect breeding ground for ... breeding. The problem, however, is that it is also a perfect breeding ground for infection, as it is a moist and warm environment for both the survival of sperm and germs. The vagina is also perilously close to the anus, making it all too easy for bacteria to spread to it.

Vaginitis, inflammation of the vagina, can be caused by various organisms such as fungus *(Candida albicans)*, bacteria *(Gardnerella)*, or protozoan *(Trichomonas vaginalis)*. Candida, or yeast, is the most common cause of vaginal infections. Yeast infections frequently result from the use of antibiotics, which may help kill the "bad" bacteria, but also knock off the "good" bacteria that are important in preventing fungal growth.

Vaginitis can also result from stress; poor diet; chemical irritation (from douches, spermicides, or feminine hygiene sprays); not enough lubrication during intercourse; and drugs or hormones that throw the system out of balance. Women who are pregnant become more susceptible to yeast infections.

Not all vaginal discharges indicate vaginitis. Some vaginal discharges are normal and healthy secretions that are an integral part of the body's own self-cleaning and self-healing functions. If, however, the discharge is profuse, smelly, or discolored, or if you feel like you have become a cottage cheese factory, you may have vaginitis. These symptoms usually suggest some type of acute, self-limiting infection; however, they can also be signs of more serious ailments, so it is recommended that you seek medical attention.

Here are some strategies that may leave you only scratching your head wondering why you didn't consider reading this book earlier.

Get cultured. Eating yogurt and douching with it (two or three tablespoons in a quart of warm water) is often effective for yeast infections (it is not effective for other vaginal infections). Make certain to use only unsweetened and unflavored yogurt, and when douching, do so just prior to going to sleep. You can also apply the yogurt directly to the outer genital area for relief of irritation. As an alternative, *Lactobacillus acidophilus* tablets can either be eaten, or the ½ teaspoon of the liquid form can inserted in the vagina to inhibit yeast imbalance. Don't douche more than once a day, and don't douche at all if you're pregnant.

A vinegar soak. Vinegar can acidify the vagina and make it less hospitable to infection. Douche with it (two tablespoons per pint of water) and/or take a bath in it (½ cup in a bathtub). Some people also place two tablespoons of green clay in the water. Don't douche more than once a day.

Herbal strategies. Goldenseal and Oregon grape contain berberine, which has a direct effect on various bacteria. Use in an herbal douche. Make a tea with one teaspoon of the powder from one or both of these herbs in one quart of water; let the water cool down before you douche with it. Tea tree oil *(Maleluca alternifolia)* is also effective for various types of vaginitis; bathe the genital area with it.

Don't overdouche yourself. Douching can wash away friendly bacteria and make a woman more susceptible to infection. Don't do it more than once a day for a week. During noninfected times, it is generally not necessary to douche.

A stinking rose for a red lady. Garlic, the stinking rose, has both antifungal and antibacterial actions. There are numerous ways to use this herb. If you're brave enough, you can eat a clove of it several times a day. Ideally, it is best to chop up fresh garlic, and let it sit for 15 minutes before eating or cooking it. This oxidation significantly increases the beneficial components in garlic. For more sociable types, take odorless garlic capsules.

The A-team. Vitamin A and beta-carotene are important for the health of epithelial tissues, such as the vaginal mucosa. Take 25,000 IU or 200,000 IU of beta-carotene per day.

C for yourself. Vitamin C helps reduce the bacteria-destroying activity of white blood cells and improves connective tissue integrity, which reduces the spread of infection. Take 500–1,000 mg every four hours.

Zinc for yourself. There is some evidence that women with recurrent vaginitis have low zinc levels in their blood. Try taking a zinc supplement (15 mg/day).

Don't wipe yourself out. When you wipe after using the bathroom, be certain to wipe from front to back. When wiping from back to front, you may accidentally spread bacteria from the anus into the vagina.

To sex or not to sex. If having sex hurts, don't do it. It's best to avoid intercourse when you're infected. If you still wish to have sex, use vegetable oil or some other natural means of lubrication. If a woman is having recurrent infections, her partner should get himself checked out to make certain that he is not a carrier. In the meantime, he should use a condom.

Haircut therapy. Some women, especially those who live in hot and humid climates, find that cutting their pubic hair shorter reduces vaginal moistness and helps to prevent vaginitis. However, keep the curling iron away.

Go natural. Sleep without underwear to let your vagina breathe freely. At other times, wear loose, natural-fiber clothing, especially cotton underwear. Avoid wearing pantyhose too frequently since it doesn't allow proper ventilation to the vagina, and avoid sitting around in a wet bathing suit.

Smell natural. Avoid deodorant tampons or deodorant sanitary napkins, scented douches, scented or dyed toilet paper, bubble baths, and products containing chemicals with which your vagina may come into contact. Some women are also sensitive to certain detergents. If you suspect you may be, change whatever detergent you are using to wash your clothes (purer brands are available in most health food stores). Some women even have a problem when using colored toilet paper.

Change pads more frequently. Tampons can be breeding grounds for infections once they become stained with blood. Also, some tampons are so absorbent that they interfere with normal vaginal secretions, thus making the woman more susceptible to infection. Consider using sanitary napkins whenever possible.

Get in hot and cold water. Alternate hot and then cold water in a Sitz bath. Ten minutes in each is sufficient.

Don't get too sweet. Although you may love sweets, so does yeast. A higher blood sugar level results from eating sweets and drinking alcohol. Avoid these items, and eat a healthy, well-balanced diet of fresh, unrefined foods.

Psyche yourself out. Psychological stress can directly affect hormones and make a woman more susceptible to infection. Any illness is stressful, and if you can relax so that the body can work its own self-healing wonders, you may become healthier sooner. Meditation is much more effective in achieving health-promoting stages of relaxation than just lying back and watching television. Don't just sit there ... relax.

A Note about Using Homeopathic Medicines

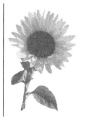

Although most readers of this book are familiar with nutritional supplements and herbal remedies, fewer people are familiar with homeopathic medicines and how best to use them.

Homeopathic medicines are safe and effective natural remedies for various acute and chronic health problems. There is, however, no single homeopathic medicine that is right for everybody's headache, allergy, flu, or whatever. For most effective results, these medicines need to be individually prescribed based on the individual's unique pattern of symptoms.

This book provides basic information on common homeopathic remedies for numerous ailments, but it is recommended that you also use one or more of the homeopathic guidebooks mentioned in the bibliography. In addition to providing more detailed information about the homeopathic remedies mentioned in this book, these books will provide you with information about other homeopathic medicines that may be indicated in treating your unique pattern of symptoms.

Depending upon the intensity of the pain, the homeopathic remedies should be taken as often as once every 30 minutes for extreme pain, or as little as three times a day when only mild discomfort is experienced. Most commonly, people take them every four hours while awake.

Quite distinct from vitamins, homeopathic medicines should not be taken every day or for prolonged periods. People usually do not need to take them for more than two to four days. Most people notice some improvement in health within 24 hours. If you do not notice any changes in your symptoms within 48 hours, you should consider taking a different homeopathic remedy.

You should not take homeopathic remedies after the pain or discomfort is gone. These medicines stimulate the body's own healing abilities and are like a spark in lighting a fire; once the fire has been lit, it is not necessary to continue to give it sparks. In fact, continued dosing of a remedy sometimes results in symptoms of overdose (which vary according to the specific medicine taken), which will stop shortly after doses are no longer taken.

If a homeopathic medicine works temporarily but the symptoms continue to return over the long run, a deeper-acting homeopathic remedy is probably needed. Professional homeopathic care is recommended in such instances. Homeopaths are trained to prescribe "constitutional medicines"—that is, homeopathic medicines that are individually chosen to treat the person's totality of symptoms according to their genetic disposition, their history of acute and chronic illness, and their physical and psychological state.

Homeopathic medicines come in different strengths. The most common potencies for the general public are 3, 6, 12, and 30. These numbers refer to the number of times a substance has been diluted and then shaken. Minerals and other substances that are not water-soluble are sequentially triturated or ground up and diluted with a lactose powder. When a substance has been diluted 1:10 (1 part of the substance to 10 parts distilled water), there is an "X" after the number ("X" in Roman numerals stands for 10). When a substance has been diluted 1:100, there is a "C" after the number ("C" in Roman numerals stands for 100).

For instance, when a medicine has been diluted 1:10 twelve times (with vigorous shaking between each dilution), the medicine is considered a 12X. If this medicine was diluted 1:100 twelve times, it is considered a 12C. Both of these types of potencies are effective. When recommendations for a specific potency (such as 6 or 30) are made in this book, no differentiation is made between "X" and "C" potencies because homeopaths do not generally consider the effects of these two potencies to be significantly different.

Despite using such small doses of medicines, more than 200 years of homeopathic practice has confirmed that the more a homeopathic substance has been potentized, the longer and deeper it acts and the fewer doses are needed.

After the medicines have been diluted and shaken, they are made with lactose or sucrose into pills, pellets, or globules (cake sprinkle size). The number of pills to be taken per dose is always listed on the bottle or in its packaging. Generally, two to eight pills are adequate. Some homeopathic medicines from the plant kingdom are made into tinctures (alcohol-based solutions), ointments, lotions, gels, or creams.

There are several important factors to keep in mind when taking homeopathic remedies to ensure their effectiveness. For best results, it is recommended to:

- avoid touching the medicines with your hands (when taking them, pour the pills into a clean spoon or inside the bottle's cap);
- place the medicine under your tongue and let it dissolve;
- avoid eating food or drinking anything but water for 15 minutes before or after taking a homeopathic medicine, but do not delay taking a dose if illness or injury begins immediately after eating or drinking (gum, toothpaste, and cough drops should also be avoided);
- keep the medicines in a place where there are no strong odors or bright lights.

The most economical way to purchase homeopathic medicines is to get a homeopathic medicine kit, which is available on a mail-order basis and through select health food stores.

Recommended Resources

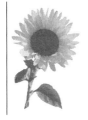

I hope that this book has inspired you to learn more about natural healing. Some of the following resources provide an overview of natural healing concepts, while others recommend specific strategies for healing. This list is not meant to be complete; it consists of those publications that I have personally read, appreciated, and used.

General Health

Achterberg, Jeanne. *Imagery in Healing.* Boston: Shambhala, 1985.

Becker, Robert O. *Cross Currents: The Perils of Electropollution, the Promise of Electromedicine.* New York: Jeremy Tarcher, 1990.

Brown, Chip. *Afterwards, You're a Genius.* New York: Riverhead, 1998.

Castleman, Michael. *Cold Cures.* New York: Fawcett, 1987.

———. *Nature Cures.* Emmaus, PA: Rodale, 1996.

Dadd, Debra Lynn. *Nontoxic, Natural, and Earthwise.* New York: Jeremy Tarcher, 1990.

Dossey, Larry. *Healing Words.* New York: HarperSanFrancisco, 1993.

Gach, Michael Reed. *Acupressure's Potent Points.* New York: Bantam, 1990.

Gerber, Richard. *Vibrational Medicine.* Santa Fe: Bear and Company, 1988.

Goldberg, Burton (ed.) *Alternative Medicine: The Definitive Guide.* Tiburon, CA: Future Medicine, 1993.

Gordon, Rena, Barbara Cable Nienstedt, and Wilbert M. Gesler. *Alternative Therapies: Expanding Options in Health Care.* New York: Springer, 1998.

Hoffman, Ronald. *Seven Weeks to a Settled Stomach.* New York: Simon and Schuster, 1990.

B. K. S. Iyengar. *Light on Yoga.* New York: Schocken, 1979.

Klein, Allen. *The Healing Power of Humor.* New York: Jeremy Tarcher, 1989.

Laux, Marcus, and Christine Conrad. *Natural Woman, Natural Menopause.* New York: HarperCollins, 1997.

Lerner, Michael. *Choices in Healing.* Cambridge, MA: MIT Press, 1994.

Murray, Michael T. *Natural Alternatives to Over-the-Counter and Prescription Drugs.* New York: William Morrow, 1994.

Murray, Michael T. and Joseph Pizzorno. E*ncyclopedia of Natural Medicine.* Rocklin, CA: Prima, 1991.

Nesse, Randolph M. and George C. Williams. *Why We Get Sick: The New Science of Darwinian Medicine.* New York: Times Books, 1994.

Ornish, Dean. *Dr. Dean Ornish's Program for Reversing Heart Disease.* New York: Random House, 1990.

Ornstein, Robert and David Sobel, *Healthy Pleasures.* New York: Addison Wesley, 1990.

Payer, Lynn. *Medicine and Culture.* New York: Henry Holt, 1988.

——. *Disease Mongers.* New York: John Wiley, 1992.

Prevention editors. *The Doctor's Book of Home Remedies.* Emmaus, PA, Rodale, 1990.

Schmidt, Michael. *Healing Childhood Ear Infections.* Berkeley: North Atlantic, 1996.

Ullman, Dana. *The Steps to Healing: Wisdom from the Sages, the Rosemarys, and the Times.* Carlsbad, CA: Hay House, 1999.

Weil, Andrew. *Health and Healing.* Boston: Houghton Mifflin, 1983.

——. *Natural Health, Natural Medicine.* Boston: Houghton Mifflin, 1990.

Whitmont, Edward C. *The Alchemy of Healing.* Berkeley: North Atlantic, 1994.

Nutrition

Balch, James F. and Phyllis A. *Prescription for Nutritional Healing.* New York: Avery, 1997.

Carper, Jean. *The Food Pharmacy.* New York: Bantam, 1988.

Davies, Stephen and Alan Stewart. *Nutritional Medicine.* New York: Avon, 1987.

Gallagher, John. *Good Health with Vitamins and Minerals.* New York: Summit, 1990.

Janson, Michael. *The Vitamin Revolution.* Greenville, NH: Arcadia, 1996.

McDougall, John A. *The McDougall Program for Women.* New York: Dutton, 1999.

Murray, Michael T. *Encyclopedia of Nutritional Supplements.* Rocklin, CA: Prima, 1996.

Null, Gary. *The Complete Guide to Sensible Eating.* New York: Four Walls Eight Windows, 1990.

Reuben, Carolyn and Joan Priestly. *Essential Supplements for Women.* New York: Pedigree, 1989.

Robbins, John. *Diet for a New America.* Walpole, NH: Stillpoint, 1987.

Robbins, John. *Reclaiming Our Health.* Tiburon, CA: HJ Kramer, 1996.

Homeopathic Medicine

Chappell, Peter. *Emotional Healing with Homeopathy.* Berkeley: North Atlantic, 2003.

Cummings, Stephen and Dana Ullman. *Everybody's Guide to Homeopathic Medicines.* New York: Jeremy Tarcher/Putnam, 1997.

Hershoff, Asa. *Homeopathic Remedies.* New York: Avery, 1999.

Reichenberg-Ullman, Judyth, and Robert Ullman, *Prozac-Free: Homeopathic Medicines for Depression, Anxiety, and Other Mental and Emotional Problems.* Berkeley: North Atlantic, 2002.

Ullman, Dana. *Homeopathy A–Z.* Carlsbad: Hay House, 1999.

——. *Consumers Guide to Homeopathy.* New York: Jeremy Tarcher/Putnam, 1995.

——. *Homeopathic Medicines for Children and Infants.* New York: Jeremy Tarcher/Putnam, 1991.

——. *Discovering Homeopathy: Medicine for the 21st Cen*tury. Berkeley: North Atlantic, 1991.

Herbs

Blumenthal, Mark, et al. (editors). *The ABC Clinical Guide to Herbs.* New York: Thieme, 2003.

Blumenthal, Mark, et al. (editors). *The Complete German Commission E Monographs.* Austin: American Botanical Council, 1998.

Brown, Don. *Herbal Prescriptions for Better Health.* Rocklin, CA: Prima, 1996.

Castleman, Michael. *The Healing Herbs.* Emmaus, PA: Rodale, 1991.

McQuade Crawford, Amanda. *Herbal Remedies for Women.* Rocklin, CA: Prima, 1997.

PDR for Herbal Medicines. Montvale, NJ: Medical Economics, 1999.

Murray, Michael. *The Healing Power of Herbs.* Rocklin: Prima, 1995.

Tierra, Michael. *The Way of Herbs.* New York: Pocket, 1990.

Wormwood, Valerie Ann. *The Fragrant Mind.* Novato, CA: New World Library, 1996.

Magazines, Newsletters, and Journals

Alternative and Complementary Therapies. 2 Madison Ave., Larchmont, NY 10538.

Alternative Therapies in Health and Medicine. 169 Saxony Road #104, Encinitas, CA 92024

Dr. Andrew Weil's Self Healing. 42 Pleasant St., Watertown, MA 02472.

Focus on Alternative and Complementary Therapies (FACT). Pharmaceutical Press, 1 Lambeth High St., London SE1 7NJ, UK.

Health Facts. 130 MacDougal St., New York, NY 10012.

HerbalGram. 620 Manor Road, Austin, TX 78723.

Homeopathy Today, 801 N. Fairfax #301, Alexandria, VA 22314.

Journal of Alternative and Complementary Therapies. 2 Madison Ave., Larchmont, NY 10538.

Let's Live. 11050 Santa Monica Blvd., Los Angeles, CA 90025.

Natural Health. P.O. Box 37474, Boone, IA 50037.

Townsend Letter for Doctors. 911 Tyler St., Port Townsend, WA 98368.

U.C. Berkeley Wellness Letter. P.O. Box 420148, Palm Coast, FL 32142.

Yoga Journal. P.O. Box 51151, Boulder, CO 80322.

Dana is interested in hearing about the insights and experiences that you have after reading this book. Feel free to contact him:

Dana Ullman, M.P.H.
2124 Kittredge St., Box Q
Berkeley, CA. 94704
Mail@homeopathic.com
www.homeopathic.com